CREATION
Health

Secrets for Feeling Fit and Living Long

Des Cummings, Jr., Ph.D.
with Monica P. Reed, M.D.

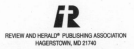

REVIEW AND HERALD® PUBLISHING ASSOCIATION
HAGERSTOWN, MD 21740

General Editor: Todd Chobotar
Edited by Gerald Wheeler and Andy Nash
Copyedited by Jocelyn Fay and James Cavil
Cover design by PierceCreative
Typeset: Bembo 11/13

ISBN 0-8280-1808-1

Contents

To order, call 1-800-765-6955.

For more information on Review and Herald® products, please visit us on the Web at www.reviewandherald.org

Bibliographic notations for the scientific studies referred to in this book are available at www. CREATIONHealth.com.

Foreword

What a pleasure to write an introduction to this inspiring and wise book! As a cardiologist, researcher, husband, and father, I have emphasized the message so thoughtfully elucidated in CREATION Health in both my personal and professional life. But it wasn't always this way.

My odyssey toward understanding the profound linkage between daily lifestyle decisions, spirituality, and good health got off to a slow start. As a lifelong athlete, walker, and runner, I entered Harvard Medical School in the fall of 1975 filled with the desire to make the world a less fat, more fit place to live. After all, I reasoned, who could resist the message to take better care of themselves!

Four years later I emerged with a very different worldview. I had been immersed in the wonders of high-tech medicine and became convinced that good medicine and great doctors were the keys to good health. Next I entered one of the toughest residency programs in the country at Massachusetts General Hospital and ultimately pursued a career as a cardiologist. I was determined to fight disease with all the high-tech tools available to modern medicine.

Trained as a hammer, I went looking for nails! I performed heart catheterizations, took care of patients in an advanced coronary-care unit, and began to edit the major intensive-care unit textbook in the world.

For 10 years I pursued this high-tech approach to medicine and health, but slowly it began to dawn on me that there had to be a better way. Often in the cardiac catheterization laboratory I felt like the farmer grabbing the tail of the horse after it had escaped the barn. As we battled complex diseases in desperately ill people, increasingly I found myself wanting to close the barn door before the horse got out—to prevent disease rather than trying to fix it once it was established.

I started a research laboratory and began studying the role of exercise, nutrition, mind-body connections, and weight management in good health, then communicated our findings to audiences around the world. In this context I discovered Celebration Health and the new vision of health it embodied. In 1999 I received an invitation to start an executive health assessment program at this facility that would incorporate both health and healing. We based our program on a concept drawn from the paradigm of CREATION so beautifully described in this book. The "Five Pillars of Good Health" consists of disease prevention or early detection, sound nutrition, regular physical activity, mind-body interactions, and the proper use of medicines and supplements to maximize health and healing. Four years later I am happy to report that Rippe Health Assessment has become the fastest growing executive health assessment program in the United States.

No one is more qualified to explain the CREATION principle of good health than Des Cummings. He served as the driving force and first CEO of Celebration Health. Every day Des emphasized to everyone involved the importance of **C**hoice, **R**est, **E**nvironment, **A**ctivity, **T**rust, **I**nterpersonal Relations, **O**utlook, and **N**utrition as our guiding principles—a vision he now shares with you in this inspiring book.

Earlier I mentioned my professional odyssey toward a deeper view of health and healing, but my journey had one more stop, a deeply personal one.

Nine years ago I fell in love with and married a beautiful woman, Stephanie Hart Rippe. Although both of us were rather late in our lives to start a family, we both wanted children. Because of our ages and some medical issues we feared we could never have a family, but we were determined to try. Often we held hands and prayed. We didn't ask God for a child, only that His will be done—and promised our commitment to be good parents.

At first we weren't successful and even became discouraged, but eventually our prayers were answered, and we were blessed with a little girl—Hart Elizabeth Rippe. As a physician, I had the thrill of actually delivering our first child. As I held her in my hands and looked into her face, I knew that I had touched the face of God.

Now, three daughters later (Jaelin, Devon, and Jamie), I am surrounded by more love and meaning than I ever dreamed would enter my life. This personal miracle for Stephanie and me convinced me that anyone who doesn't believe in a divine Creator has never truly pondered the miracles of birth or life itself.

This book, *CREATION Health,* is about these miracles—and the power that each of us has to live each day fully and with meaning. Each of us has the ability to create good health and healing in our own lives and the lives of those around us—to see and experience the miracles that surround us every day. I urge you to read *CREATION Health,* study its principles, and pass it along to friends!

James M. Rippe, M.D.
Founder and Director, Rippe Health Assessment
Florida Hospital Celebration Health
Author of *Fit Over Forty* and *Fitness Walking*

Acknowledgments

The Adventist Health System was founded by visionary leaders who were committed to helping people get well and stay well. This commitment led to a study of the principles of health and healing contained in this book. Millions of people have adopted these principles. As a result they have dramatically improved their health and lengthened their lives.

For more than 100 years the Adventist Health System has shared these principles in the communities that we serve.

This book is based on the premise that the model for health is embedded in the Creation story. This model can be summarized in eight principles that form the basis of CREATION Health. By applying these eight principles that God built into the Garden of Eden we can experience "optimum vitality." My wife, Mary Lou, has helped me to actualize these principles in my life and demonstrate how they can be designed into a care model for The Women's Center at Celebration Health.

My deepest professional appreciation is also due to my coauthor, Monica Reed, M.D., who implemented these principles as the first medical director of the Women's Center at Celebration Health. Her work on this book has been invaluable.

My work at Florida Hospital has been among the most rewarding experiences of my life. I would like to thank Tom Werner and Don Jernigan, Ph.D., for their unwavering support and encouragement. Without their visionary leadership Celebration Health and the CREATION Health model wouldn't be what they are today.

Lars Houmann and Brian Paradis have had a lasting impact on my life and helped me to shape many of the ideas in this book. We worked together for more than three incredible years to implement these principles at Celebration Health.

I owe a special debt of thanks to the team who helped create the vision of the CREATION Health principles. My sincere thanks are due to Ted Hamilton, M.D., who wrote the original philosophy statement; Dick Tibbits, who coached the health professionals in implementing it; and Kevin Edgerton, who developed the communications materials to popularize it. The catalyst for much of the work on this book was an eight-part television series that Florida Hospital embarked on with Mark Finley, director and speaker of the *It Is Written* program. Many of those involved in the production of the CREATION Health series are excellent writers and provided material for structuring this book. In particular I would like to thank Steve Mosley, Dick Duerksen, Todd Chobotar, Sherri Flynt, Susan Sipprell, Simon Lia, Stacy Nelson, and Lorraine Zima-Lenon.

A number of people actively participated in researching and shaping this manuscript in its early form. For this I am indebted to Nick Hall, M.D., Andy Nash, Amanda Sauder, and Lillian Boyd.

1

The Original Formula
for Feeling Great

*"You can never have too many friends
or too much honey."*

—*Winnie the Pooh*

This could well be the most important book you will read this year. It will help you to experience life at its very best and find new energy and peace. The ideas you will find here could turn your whole life upside down—*for the better!*

Now, before you get nervous, let me tell you what this book won't do. It won't demand that you go on a broccoli-only diet, that you run 12 miles each day, or that you start taking 10-minute naps each hour.

I would love to tell you that *the secret of optimum health* is eating an ice-cream bar every afternoon, but this book is not about fads or extremes—it's about learning a new way to think about your life.

Sound simple? It is—and it isn't. The concept is simple—eight easy-to-remember steps to a new life. But, like everything good, the process demands commitment, energy, and time. Yet it will bring rewards far beyond anything the stock market has ever offered.

You can have a better life! *The best life!*

THIS IS FOR YOU!

No matter what level of health you may have, the principles in this book can take you even higher. Should you not be happy with your present health, this book can get you feeling and looking great.

And if you are feeling pretty good but could use a little energy boost, *CREATION Health* will lead you to new ways of increasing your vitality and adding a brighter sparkle to your eye.

CREATION Health will add new certainty to a teenager's step. For those entering the 50s or 60s or 70s (or better!) this book offers practical solutions for making every day a better day.

Sound unbelievable?

Read on and you will become a believer, a model of what life ought to be.

PERSONAL STORIES

This is not a book of esoteric psychotransformational concepts and giant words. *CREATION Health* is about people and their stories, about individual tales of change, improvement, new energy, and peace.

You'll encounter a chaplain who has turned his life around through becoming physically active. You'll meet a lawyer who learned to slow down for rest and in the process found his family. And you'll read the story of a cancer researcher who got cancer himself, and how his interpersonal relationships saved him. Through these stories and more, you'll learn the principles that can change your life as well.

When people decide to alter their lives—when they make personal commitments to make wiser choices, to enjoy adequate rest, to celebrate the best in their environment, and more—amazing things happen.

This book will introduce you to new friends who have moved beyond depression, who have lost weight, who have fixed broken relationships, and who can finally wake up without fear.

No, these are not stories of people who bought into "before and after" newspaper advertisements for miracle cures. They are accounts of men and women who decided they wanted to experience complete health—mentally, physically, spiritually, and so-cially—and who followed the CREATION Health principles to get there.

HOW THIS BOOK WILL CHANGE YOU

First, it will inspire you that there is a better way to life and that you can get there!

Then it will teach you how to master the eight most powerful principles for improving every part of your life.

You will discover the scientific research behind each of the eight principles—carefully designed stud-ies, performed by major universities and institutes—that point the way to enjoying the best health possible.

Reliable medical experts will share simple life-improvement tools you can use *today*.

You will learn the best ways to eat, exercise, and create a balanced healing environment in your life.

And you will be inspired to join others in making a commitment to change for the better.

WHERE **CREATION** HEALTH CAME FROM

It's a long story, so we've placed the whole background on a special Internet Web site: www.CREATIONHealth.com. But let me give you a quick summary.

The Florida Hospital medical team discovered the eight principles of CREATION Health while working with the Walt Disney Corporation to design the "healthiest town in America"—Celebration, Florida. Florida Hospital Celebration Health, our hospital in the town of Celebration, models the CREATION Health principles in its architecture, its medical care, its fitness center, and its customer service. We have found that following the CREATION Health principles does more than change lives—it also transforms the way we do business. *For the better!*

Sorry to give you such a tiny bit of history here, but please visit the Web site for the full story.

CREATION HEALTH, WHAT IS IT?

God loves giving good gifts. It's been that way since the dawn of time. At the creation of the world God made a spectacular planet brimming with life— flying, swimming, crawling, waddling, growing, blooming life. In the center of it all was a garden called Eden, a haven He planted as a gift for His first two children, Adam and Eve. Along with their new garden home, one of the first and finest gifts that God gave them was abundant, full health—physical health, mental health, social health, and spiritual health. By examining CREATION Health, God's original Eden design for His children, we learn much about feeling fit and living long today. The principles God established for wellness are timeless.

Full health is more than the absence of disease and its symptoms; it is God's moment-by-moment empowering to become more like Him—In His Image!

After reading and re-reading the Genesis accounts of Creation, and after spending many hours considering God's plans for our health, the Florida Hospital Mission Team chose to use CREATION Health as an easy-to-remember acronym for full health. The letters of the acronym stand for:

Choice
Rest and Relaxation
Environment
Activity
Trust in Divine Power
Interpersonal Relationships
Outlook
Nutrition

In this book we've taken these principles and transformed them into a handful of easy-to-follow *life recipes*. Embracing the CREATION Health prescription can restore health, happiness, balance, and joy. These eight principles are the Creator's gift to help us experience life as He designed us to live it.

WHAT'S NEXT?

Before you turn to Chapter 2 and begin the next step on our CREATION Health journey, let me share one more insight about health and wellness.

All of us want to live without sickness, to have healthy legs, sharp eyes, and quick minds. We want to be healed from everything unhealthy, and we would prefer not having to worry about cancer, accidents, and aging. Desiring to be healthy is good.

But CREATION Health is about *wellness,* and *wellness* is more than health. *Wellness* is being mentally fit, physically robust, spiritually vital, and socially comfortable. It is being able to face accidents, aging, and illness with a positive outlook. Most of all, it is trusting that God has a "better idea" for living, and that He is eager to help us experience full Life—*as He created us to live it!*

Welcome to CREATION Health, God's prescription for living.

2

Take Charge
of Your Health

The "C" in CREATION Health stands for *Choice*. We are what we choose. Some of our choices are important to daily life, but have no moral impact. However, many contain moral challenges, powerful options that could change the direction of life. That's where God comes in, standing ready to help us make decisions that will draw us closer to Him and develop His characteristics in us.

Our choices transform who we are and shape how we influence those around us. They make us either more like God or more like His enemy. But in each situation God is there, offering all the resources necessary so we can make the healthiest possible choice. As He knows, healthy choices make healthy people.

SCIENTIFIC SUPPORT FOR *CHOICE*

Researchers at Yale University found that when people have a choice in their medical treatment, they respond better to it. At the time of the study, two approaches were commonly used to treat ulcers, and the doctor usually decided whether medication or a restricted diet would be best. Doctors Rodin and Langer used a different approach. They allowed the patients to be a part of the decision-making process. They described each treatment option along with the pros and cons. Then the patients decided which they wanted. Regardless of whether they selected the medication or diet-based treatment, those who had a choice always did better than those who did exactly the same thing just because the doctor ordered it.

When we make choices, we are taking responsibility and exerting a degree of control. This is a major determinant of how disease progresses. Scientists have shown that even laboratory animals respond differently depending upon whether or not they are able to control their circumstances. When exposed to adversity, animals that are able to make a choice to stop the stress are far less likely to suffer from disease compared with the animals that are helpless. The same is true of people. Sometimes circumstances may leave little in your control. But you can always decide what you will focus upon and the attitude you adopt toward it.

Drugs used to manage chronic pain can become addictive. For that reason physicians must carefully control and mentor the use of such drugs. However, it was also recognized that the uncertainty about whether the medication would be available when needed was making the pain worse for some patients. In a controversial decision, some hospitals allowed patients to administer their own pain medication whenever they needed it. Instead of using more as expected, the patients actually took less medication. Nothing new had been done to alleviate the pain, but now patients no longer worried about whether the nurse heard their request or whether the drug would be made available. Just having the choice was enough to make the pain more tolerable.

TAKE CHARGE OF YOUR HEALTH

A few years ago a young physician walked into Celebration Health—the "hospital of the twenty-first century" created by Florida Hospital in partnership with the Walt Disney Corporation. Severely over-weight, he was starting to experience heart problems. Because his family had a history of heart disease, he was naturally concerned. He and his wife had just had a baby, and absolutely adoring his little girl, he wanted to be around for her.

When he started having heart symptoms, he decided, as a medical doctor, that it was time to take charge of his own health. So he came to our fitness center and started an exercise program. In time he lost more than 40 pounds and began to change his entire health future.

"Put first things first, and we get second things thrown in. Put second things first, and we lose both first and second things."

—C. S. Lewis

One day at the fitness center I bumped into him. "Man!" I said. "You look totally different. What in the world's happened to you?"

"I've gotta tell you," he said. "One evening I had my little daughter crawl up in my lap. For the first time in my life I realized that I not only wanted to watch my children grow up, but to see my grandchildren grow up as well. And I knew that if I was going to do that, I had to choose a different destiny than some of my other family members. I had to retain my health, and I had to make healthy choices.

"At first," he continued, "it was very hard work. But now it's become a lifestyle for me. I'm eating different, I'm living different, and I'm feeling different. And I believe that I will see my grandchildren and enjoy their company as well as I do my own children."

THE IMPORTANCE OF CHOICE

Choice is our greatest asset and a very precious gift. Holocaust survivor Viktor E. Frankl wrote, "The last of human freedoms [is] . . . to choose one's own way."

Our ability to make decisions is one of the most important gifts that we human beings have. Ever notice how hopeless people feel when they don't have a choice. They feel like victims, that there is no point in trying to change their situation. Understanding that you *do* have a choice and that you always *will* have, no matter what the circumstances, is a highly empowering thought.

How important are the choices we make?

Some choices, such as what color to wear to work, have no lasting consequences. However, other decisions may result in outcomes that we have to live with for the rest of our lives. Studies show that many of the conditions that we're dying from today—heart disease, hypertension, obesity, diabetes, and certain cancers—are the direct result of lifestyle choices. In many cases they are diseases of overeating and under-activity. Many of these lifestyle diseases—perhaps as high as 80 to 90 percent of them—could be eliminated with healthier lifestyle choices.

When it comes to our physical health, then, our decisions *do* make a difference.

Choice From the Start

God gave us choices from the very beginning, despite the fact that He knew that we might not always make the best ones.

In the Garden of Eden Adam and Eve had a wealth of healthy things to choose from. Fruits and vegetables to nourish them, physical work to strengthen their bodies, and a relationship with the Creator to feed their souls. But God also gave them another choice—the tree of the knowledge of good and evil. "The Lord God took the man and put him in the Garden of Eden to work it and take care of it. And the Lord God commanded the man, 'You are free to eat from any tree in the garden; but you must not eat from the tree of the knowledge of good and evil, for when you eat of it you will surely die" (Genesis 2:15-17).

The tree represented all the unhealthy choices that Adam and Eve could make. All the decisions that could hurt them physically, spiritually, socially, and emotionally. Making this one choice—to eat from that tree—would result in a life that would be less than what God wanted for them. And in the end, the consequence would be death. It might be a quick death, or it might be a slow death. But the end result was the same.

God didn't hide this choice from our first human parents. He didn't pretend that it didn't exist. Instead,

He created them as free moral agents with the ability to choose to follow His plan for their lives because it was the best way to live, not because anything forced them to do so.

Choice is at the very heart of the story of the Garden of Eden. And it's at the very heart of the Creator's wonderful plan for our health.

WE HAVE A CHOICE

The principle that lies at the foundation of the CREATION model of health is simple: choice. The Creator loudly and clearly declares that you have a choice. No matter your genetics or the condition of your environment, you can follow a healthy lifestyle. You can participate in your own healing, be part of the process of restoration. God has made you the steward of your own body.

Because God loves us, however, He doesn't just let us attempt to make healthy choices on our own. He promises to help us in our decisions. In effect, to choose *with* us. God gives us the understanding and strength to make consistently healthy choices. The Creator acts as a re-creator inside us through His Spirit.

The apostle Paul relied on God's promises to do just that. You can see it throughout his letters in the New Testament. "I can do all things through Christ who strengthens me," he wrote (Philippians 4:13, NKJV).

I can do all things. Nothing is impossible. Now, *that's* confidence. That's a positive attitude. Paul believed this because he trusted in the God who was working inside him. He believed in the God who will strengthen every one of us through His Spirit.

That's why we can say that the first principle of CREATION Health is choice. And this decision involves living life as God intended.

> *"Wherever God's finger points,*
> *His hand will clear a way."*
>
> —L. B. Cowman

But remember, God still surrounded Adam and Eve with love even after they made unhealthy choices. Look at what happened when they ate the forbidden fruit—when they began to realize what their decision would cost them and were overwhelmed with guilt. "And [Adam and Eve] heard the sound of the Lord God walking in the garden in the cool of the day, and Adam and his wife hid themselves from the presence of the Lord God among the trees of the garden" (Genesis 3:8, NKJV).

Notice something rather amazing in this description. God Himself was walking in the Garden, looking for His children. Although He knew what had happened, He still wanted to continue the relationship. He didn't turn His back on them. The biblical account depicts Adam and Eve as the ones who are hiding. After He searches them out, the Creator has to inform the couple about the consequences of their actions. But He also assures them that He still has a plan that leads to life—He still has their best interest at heart.

MAKING THE BEST CHOICES

Managing your health is a challenge, one determined by the choices that you make daily. The Health

Institute in Washington, D.C., affirms that behavior change is related to a person's view of risk, benefit, and opportunity. Will Schutz, Ph.D., in his book *Profound Simplicity,* states that to make decisions that last, you must become more aware of your options and their consequences. It is important to be honest with yourself. Do you really want change? Why? Do you understand the benefits of smart health choices? Do you recognize the risks when you don't make those choices? One of the most important factors in making wise decisions is good information. The more you read and understand about your health, the more likely you are to be willing to change.

Sometimes knowledge is not enough, nor is sheer willpower. How often have you made New Year's resolutions that fizzle and die after only one month? David Katz, M.D., M.P.H., of Yale School of Medicine, states that there has to be "a reasonable way as well." In other words, if the difficulty in making any changes outweighs your motivation, you will not alter your behavior (we've all heard stories about people not using their health club memberships because the gym is all the way across town).

The thought of making healthy changes can sound overwhelming, but it is not impossible. Choice is the foundation of a balanced, healthy life. The other seven CREATION Health principles will work only when we accept our gift of choice and use it according to God's guidance. Let me encourage you to decide every day to live the life for which God created you. Here are a few practical tips to ensure your success:

1. Choose—The first step to living a healthy, bal-

anced life is to make the decision that it is what you want. It will be an everyday choice, a commitment to live a balanced, healthy existence.

2. Notice—Once you have accepted God's prescription for living, take a look at the balance of your life. Are there areas that are keeping you from enjoying full health, aspects that you would like to bring into balance?

3. Prioritize—Look at the out-of-balance areas and choose your priorities. It would be wonderful if everything could be fixed at once, but it doesn't quite work that way. Choose one area—no more than two—for your attention. If you are out of balance in the area of rest, what choices are you willing to make to increase your rest time? If your top priority is more activity, are you willing to get up early and take a walk? Healthy changes require conscious effort, so keep them simple and realistic. This will help to remove many barriers and set you up for success.

4. Act—Once you have chosen your priorities, it's time for setting goals and taking action! Again, don't plan to bring everything into balance by this afternoon. Instead, choose realistic small-step goals that you truly *can do* today. For instance, if your goal is to eat more healthfully, a goal of "never eating chocolate cake again" probably will not work. But choosing cake only once a week may be an ideal step on the road to nutritional success. Keep your goals simple and doable and you will set your-

self up for success.

So what about it? Wouldn't you like to make healthy choices today because a wonderful Creator loves you? Right now you can start taking positive steps that will turn your life around—physically, spiritually, socially, and emotionally. You can begin a journey that will take you to a better place than you have ever imagined.

LIFE-CHANGE OPPORTUNITIES
YOU CAN BEGIN TODAY!

- ✓ Choose to stop at yellow lights, then do it!
- ✓ Choose to hold hands with someone you love, then follow through with your decision.
- ✓ Buy a mouse pad for your computer, one that says "Choose Life!" Buy a second one to place under the remote control for your TV set!
- ✓ Choose to smile every time you answer a telephone.
- ✓ Choose to read and follow a chapter of this book each week for eight life-changing weeks.

3

Getting Out
of the Fast Lane

The "R" in CREATION Health stands for *Rest*. Do you know the wonderfully sweet pleasure of leaning back and reveling in a good rest? That's the gift God gave on Creation's seventh day.

Loaded with smiles and packed with peace, rest comes as 10-minute power naps, 20-second mini-vacations, and eight hours of wonderful sleep. Regardless of its length, it offers energy for the burned-out and restoration for the broken. Rest replaces weariness, exhaustion, and fatigue with peace, energy, and hope. Maybe that's why the Creator wrapped a whole day of rest in a package called the Sabbath. Knowing that we would work hard all week, He dedicated an entire day for us to plug into His power, a time when He packs us full of Himself so we can be healthier people throughout the next week.

Rest. It's God's personal way of saying "I love you."

SCIENTIFIC SUPPORT FOR *REST*

Not all sleep is the same. Dr. Krueger at the University of Kentucky found that the immune system actually triggers the type of sleep best for healing. Called Delta or Slow Wave Sleep, it is the deep, rest-

ful sleep you need to awaken feeling refreshed and energized. During this stage of sleep the body releases
Growth Hormone. As its name implies, Growth
Hormone stimulates the growth and repair of dam-
aged tissue. It also stimulates the formation of lym-
phocytes needed to fight disease-causing microbes, an
important step in healing actually bought about by the
immune system. Consequently, it's available at just
the time you need it most—while fighting illness.
Listen to your body. When you start to feel tired, it
may be your immune system signaling the need for
healing sleep.

For every action there has to be an opposite and
equal reaction. More than a law of physics, it's a re-
quirement for optimal health. Stress is a part of daily
living and not likely to go away. While you may
have little influence over the circumstances that
cause you anguish, you can insert periods of rest and
recovery. Stress is beneficial in that it stimulates
change and growth. However, it is during periods of
recovery that the growth actually occurs. Successful
athletes make recovery an essential part of their
training, for without it muscles will never achieve
their full potential. Neither will the God-given healing systems that must perform on a daily basis to protect you from illness. Rest and recovery are the
opposite of stress. Without them you will never
achieve optimal health.

A relaxing massage could be more than just a quiet
interlude from the topsy-turvy world you seem to live
in. It may also be an essential ingredient for good
health. Dr. Tiffany Fields at the University of Miami

demonstrated that premature infants who were gently massaged several times each day grew at a faster rate, developed reflexes more rapidly, and had cognitive advantages compared with those premature infants who were not touched. Your skin is the largest organ in the body and, when touched, can release pain-countering endorphin as well as produce immune system stimulating Growth Hormone. Those seeking healing, not just pampering, now have restful massages.

GETTING OUT OF THE FAST LANE

We are an overstimulated society.

The world around us seeks to cram more and more into each 24-hour day. Businesses run at an ever-quickening pace. People phone, fax, e-mail, page, and overnight-deliver to us a flood of demands wherever we are in the world. And we have to respond in kind—just to keep up.

When we do sit down to relax, the stimulation only increases. Where once we had only 13 television stations to choose from, today 60 to 100 channels compete for our attention. And there are more on the way.

What about our nighttimes? Not much better. According to the National Sleep Foundation, more than 100 million Americans suffer from sleep deprivation. More than 40 percent of Americans sleep less than six hours a night, and as many as one in three are so sleepy during the day that it interferes with their performance and activities at least two to three days in each month. And guess what? Stress is the number one cause for poor sleep. Consider these familiar scenarios:

✓ A young stock trader exchanges a full night's sleep with fitful naps between transactions as he frantically tries to follow market activity around the world.

✓ A young mother accepts the night shift so she can take care of her children during the day. She describes her world as exhausting and speaks of sleep with the craving of a hungry beggar talking about food. But as she works what is basically an 80-hour week, she risks her health, her sanity, and her marriage. As she chases her dream of the good life, it cruelly imprisons her with a sentence of hard labor.

FINDING THE BALANCE

With each beat our hearts teach us the importance of respecting natural rhythms—the necessity to balance work and rest. During your lifetime your heart will beat 2.5 billion times and will pump more than 1 million barrels of blood throughout your body. It is important to note that between each powerful beat of your heart, it rests. This resting period allows the heart to reload—to do the work of the next beat.

Likewise, you and I need time to "reload." We need rest. The medical community understands this principle well—every day they see its effects when ignored. Overstimulated organs eventually flat-line. That means they shut down and die.

Kathy Grace, a Christian nurse in the Florida Hospital cardiac lab, compares our need for rest to the heart rhythm itself. "When we take care of patients," Kathy says, "we always give them an electrocardiogram [EKG], an electrical recording of the heart. It shows us the heart rhythm, or heartbeat, which is the very basis of what we do. I like to compare the heartbeat to how the Lord made us. Each waveform is a heartbeat, and the line that separates each beat is a time of rest. This is the way our lives work as well. We can have a very active day, and then we need a time of rest. We need sleep in order to stay healthy."

Kathy says they're constantly trying to teach their cardiac patients how to take time every day for rest, relaxation, and rejuvenation.

ISLAND OF TIME

Science, however, wasn't the first to discover the need for a cycle of rest. In fact, rest is part of the plan that our Creator gave to us at the very beginning. He established an island of time at the end of each week for spiritual and physical restoration.

The book of Genesis tells how God provided for this rest. During a six-day period God created all the living things on our planet, everything from crickets to crocodiles, from mushrooms to mangoes. He also made the first human beings.

It was an amazing week of work, and the Creator knew it. "God saw all that he had made, and it was very good" (Genesis 1:31). Everything was good indeed. We're still discovering today the awe-inspiring ways in which He designed even the tiniest of creatures—living things so small we can view them only through powerful microscopes.

But then watch what happened: "Thus the heavens and the earth were completed in all their vast array. By the seventh day God had finished the work he had been doing; so on the seventh day he rested from all his work" (Genesis 2:1, 2).

What was God doing here? Was He worn out from His work?

Not likely. Instead He was setting an example for us. He was building a rhythm of rest into our weekly cycle. This cycle is as much a part of nature as the rhythm of our hearts: beat, rest, beat, rest. God was creating an island of rest in our ocean of labor.

> *"Sabbath is a time to stop, to refrain from being seduced by our desires. To stop working, stop making money, stop spending money. See what you have. Look around. Listen to your life. Then, at the end of the day, where is the desperate yearning to consume, to shop, to buy what we do not need? It dissolves. Little by little it falls away."*
>
> —*Wayne Mueller*

He would make that clear when He gave the world His essential Ten Commandments from Mount Sinai. Among these basic moral principles is one that prescribes rest. The fourth commandment reads: "Remember the Sabbath day, to keep it holy. Six days you shall labor and do all your work, but the seventh day is the Sabbath of the Lord your God. In it you shall do no work" (Exodus 20:8–10, NKJV).

In other words, God is saying: "Great news! You don't have to work this day, and you don't have to feel guilty about it. This is a day for resting."

By the way, notice something else interesting about the weekly cycle of activity and rest. The seven-day week is the only part of our calendars that doesn't correspond to some celestial cycle. Think about it.

✓ We have the year, the time it takes the earth to orbit the sun.

✓ We have the month, the period from one full moon to the next.

✓ And we have the 24-hour day, one rotation of the earth on its axis.

But the week? Where does that come from? Nature has no seven-day cycles that repeat themselves again and again. Yet virtually everyone on earth observes a seven-day week.

Why? Because the week came to all of us from the hand of the Creator. Going back to the beginning, back to the garden, it's a direct link through time to the One who fashioned life on our planet. And at the climax of that week God rested, setting a pattern for us to rest as well.

DISCOVERING TRUE REST

Rest, of course, can come in many forms—through sleep, through relaxation, through meditation, through prayer, through worship, and even through relationships. Mainly I've found that rest is a person—and that person is Jesus Christ. Others are also discovering that same fact.

Scott: From Stress to Rest

Scott Brady, a physician who uses the CRE-

ATION Health principles in his medical practice, tells of his personal journey from stress to rest.

"My wife and I had been married about five years," he says. "Things were going well, and we had our first child. I was studying for boards, and both of us were working full-time. Then I began to develop some physical symptoms—back pain, headaches, and stomach problems. Medicines weren't able to help. I saw about six or seven physicians, had several different diagnoses, lots of X-rays, physical therapy. And it kept getting worse to the point at which I was having about 10 shots in my back every couple weeks just to be able to stand. I could sleep only two or three hours a night.

"It was really affecting our family. Soon I began to realize that it was more than just pain—that there were other things behind it: stresses and emotions I hadn't recognized. Once I began to acknowledge the emotions that were building up in me like a volcano, the pain started to go away. God became increasingly important in my life as I saw that I needed Him more and more. I needed to rest in His grace."

As Scott came to see, sometimes disease and pain aren't the result of genetics or physical factors but have their roots in emotional or spiritual problems. Recognizing these problems is the first step toward finding the rest that God intends for each of us.

Steve: Finding Space in My Life

Steve Kreitner, an attorney, is one of those successful young American professionals whose hectic schedule was taking its toll.

"I was leading a very, very busy life—sometimes putting in 70-hour weeks," he explains. "Every month or so I had a pretty bad migraine. I was in my early 30s and had never had migraines before. My life had just gotten so busy, and I was so tired that some cracks and strains were beginning to show in my relationships, including the one with my wife.

"I started to pray and to try to analyze my life and figure out what was missing. One of the first things that hit me was my schedule. I didn't have any time for rest. To me, rest is space within my life—space to step back and to reconnect with God, with my family, with my friends. To recharge my batteries and restore my enthusiasm with life and people. I really just needed to find that space in my life.

"I began making sure I got quality time with God. That happens both in the morning as well as on my Sabbath. The greatest benefit I've found by increasing the amount of rest in my life is that I'm now living more of a reflective life than a reactive one. Rather than a knee-jerk reaction to my circumstances, I take more time to determine what's really important to me."

Thousands of people like Scott and Steve are discovering that spiritual rest is a key part of healthy living. Taking time to bond with our Creator creates a peaceful center in our lives. And it's from that peaceful center that we can grow toward wholeness.

THE REST TEST

If you find yourself in situations similar to Scott and Steve, this Rest Test will help you understand the challenge and clarify your goals. Check each box that applies to you and then consider the 7 Rest Steps described on pages 38-40.

❑ Do you have to jump-start your brain with stimulants?

❑ Do you lose concentration often?

What fear symptoms do you experience daily?

❑ worry

❑ anxiety (general sense of stress)

❑ panic

What hurry disease symptoms do you experience daily?

❑ multitasking (drive, eat, talk on phone—all at same time)

❑ overcommitting yourself (trying to cram too many things into a day)

❑ crisis-driven (other people run your life; it is out of control)

❑ emotional (overreacting to small things)

What is your sleep pattern?

❑ I don't get enough sleep.

❑ I can't sleep.

Do you live a pattern of overwork?

❑ I work 60 or more hours a week.

❑ I feel guilty for neglecting my family.

❑ Others tell me that my life is out of balance.

Ask yourself these questions:

How many hours of sleep do you believe you need? _____

How are you going to reshape your priorities to achieve this goal?

How much time each day do you want to spend with God?

How are you going to reshape your priorities
to achieve this goal?

How much time each day do you want to
spend with your family?

How are you going to reshape your priorities
to achieve this goal?

How do you want to respond to God's invitation for a full day of rest each week?

How are you going to reshape your priorities
to achieve this goal?

GOD'S REST OPTION

In our stressed-out world, in which families are
increasingly falling apart and thousands visit hospital
emergency rooms each day because their stress has become a major health crisis, we desperately need the
kind of rest that God offers. Here is my paraphrase of
the famous invitation made in Matthew 11:28:
"Come unto me all you who labor to exhaustion, and
I will give you rest."

HeartMath (www.heartmath.com) is an organization begun by a group of scientists dedicated to teaching people how to gain maximum health through
getting the circulatory, respiratory, and nervous systems back into sync. Their approach is to teach simple activities you can do *right now* to bring your body
back into balance.

Take Power Breaks, HeartMath says. As little as
five minutes will make a tremendous difference in
how you feel and how well your body works.
"Breathe deeply, relax your mind with peaceful
thoughts, and pray. Such breaks will have profound

impact on your body and your performance." Research shows that "when we are in sync, blood pressure drops, stress hormones plummet, anti-aging hormones increase, clarity and calmness result." In short, you experience the benefits of rest. This is especially important when you face a crisis. It will enable you to be your best. Athletes call this being "in the zone"—the rest zone!

God's healing rest is as close as the beating of your heart. He has placed the rhythm of rest within the very pulse of your own body by giving rest in each heartbeat, in each day, and in each week. Why not step out of the fast lane and enjoy some sweet rest. Your body will bless you for it.

7 Rest Steps You Can Begin Today

1. Pray—Worry and anxiety often stand between us and real rest and health. Instead of becoming upset while waiting in traffic, talk with God. When you've had a rough day at work, tell Him. Let Him know your worries and cares. Then turn them over to Him and trust that He will take care of you. The Bible tells us in Philippians 4:6 "not to be anxious about anything, but in everything, by prayer and petition, with thanksgiving, present your requests to God."

2. Sleep—Develop a regular sleep pattern. If you are sleeping less than eight hours nightly, you are cheating yourself. Trying to catch up on sleep doesn't help. Here's how to get those restful zzz's: exercise daily; reduce caffeine in-

take, especially late in the day; reduce alcohol; avoid eating large, fatty meals late in the day that can keep you awake; adopt a relaxing bedtime routine, something that prepares you for sleep, such as a warm bubble bath or listening to soft music.

3. Breathe well—Proper breathing can help you relax. Try this: start from the very bottom of your lungs and breathe in slowly through your nose. Count slowly to five while inhaling. Then exhale through tight lips twice as long as you inhaled. Allow the head to drop toward the chest as you exhale, relaxing the back of your neck. Repeat this exercise four or five times until you notice your breathing is slowing down.

4. Imagine—Take 20-second (or much longer!) mental vacations. Wander through Yosemite National Park, walk along a white-sand Hawaiian beach, or browse in antique shops in Pennsylvania. By taking time "away" you will resettle or "resync" your mind and be able to face your day with new energy.

5. Take a vacation—We all love vacations, but hardly ever take them. The average American worker feels that his workload just doesn't allow for the luxury of a vacation. It is no wonder that we are living unhealthy, unbalanced lives because a balanced, healthy life includes regular time off. No, not just an occasional day here and there—even though those are helpful—but the "I went fishing in

the Keys for two weeks" kind of vacations. Studies show that our bodies need several days to unwind from the stress of everyday life. Then we need several days after that for true rest to occur. Start planning your next vacation, a real one without cell phones, computers, and other work. Get away. Play. Rest.

6. Laugh—The Bible book of Proverbs tells us that a cheerful heart is good medicine, but a crushed spirit dries up the bones. Another way of saying this is that laughter is the best medicine. When we laugh, especially those laughs that start in our toes and don't stop until they reach the top of our head, our blood pressure goes down, our muscles relax, and our brains release chemicals (endorphins) that make us feel better.

You can add laughter to your life in countless ways. Keep a joke or riddle book handy. Watch reruns of *I Love Lucy*, *Dick van Dyke*, or *The Three Stooges*. Go to a local pet store and watch the kittens and puppies play. Find whatever makes you laugh, then do it!

7. Rest weekly—Never forget the special rest that God created for us, the Sabbath rest when we leave behind our normal routine and spend one full day with Him and with family and friends. Spend the Sabbath reading the Bible and praying, enjoying nature, visiting a nursing home, going to church. Rest your body, your mind, and your soul.

Now, get some rest.

4

Taking Hints
From Paradise

The "E" in CREATION Health stands for *Environment*. God designed the world to perfectly match the people who would live in it. Then He handed it to us and said, "Take good care of it—for Me."

As caretakers we've discovered a special healing relationship between people and nature. Dig in your garden and be energized. Plant a row of petunias on your windowsill and be cheered. Watch a five-minute sunset and be revitalized.

We can find healing in a mockingbird's song or in walking beside the sea. There is healing on a mountain trail, in the desert sands, in a pine forest, on a rocky coast, and in a city park. Nature brings healing to the body, mind, and spirit. The Creator made it that way.

SCIENTIFIC SUPPORT FOR *ENVIRONMENT*

You probably have heard of Pavlov and his dogs. After allowing them to smell meat while listening to a bell, he discovered that the bell alone soon acquired the ability to induce salivation. The same thing can happen in your body. Just about anything in the environment can elicit an automatic response after an association has been established. Cancer patients, upon returning to the clinic where they received chemotherapy, will sometimes reexperience the side effects of the treatment even though they do not get any medication. Instead, pictures in the room, the fragrance worn by a staff member, and even the background music are responsible. This research conducted at the Sloan Kettering Memorial Hospital in New York underscores why it is essential to pay attention to anything at home or work that may affect your health. You may not make the connection, but your body can.

We will all remember where we were and what we were doing when we heard of the attack on the World Trade Towers in New York. Those who were there will do more than remember. The slightest reminder may trigger the same stress response they experienced during the attack. In the extreme, it results in a condition called Post Traumatic Stress Disorder or PTSD. Scientists have shown that the more emotion associated with an event, the more likely it will leave a permanent memory in your brain. We live among triggers of both unhealthy and healthy responses. Positive emotions will do the same thing. That's why we remember our wedding day or first time we got up on a slalom ski. For optimal health, create an environment that will remind you of the positive while removing those things that might trigger anxiety.

TAKING HINTS FROM PARADISE

Today we live in a world of never-ending changes in styles, fashions, fads, and trends. The latest crazes grow faster and fall flatter than ever before. All around us billboards, radio, television, magazines, the Internet, and more shout for our attention and beg to be noticed. The whole world demands our time and attention. As a result, many feel as though their life grows ever more stressful as they try to keep up with the constant changes.

Medical scientists are highlighting today that our environment has a significant impact on our health.

THE EDEN ENVIRONMENT

Take a moment to think about your personal environment—both at home and in your workplace. Are your surroundings cheerful and healthy? Are they places that nurture your soul and recharge your spirit? Do you feel calm and happy when you're in them? Do they provide you with comfort, offer you an opportunity for growth, and give you a sense of peace?

> *"It's a feeling of awe—of scientific awe—*
> *this feeling about the glories of the universe."*
> —*Richard Feynemann*

God knew the effect our environment would have on us. That's why He placed the first humans in the best possible surroundings. Though we can't expect to recreate the Garden of Eden, we can take away principles from it and then apply them to our own situations—enriching our homes and enlivening our workplaces by lessons learned from the natural world. The closer we come to making our personal environments like the original garden

43

home, the more of its benefits we will experience.

Let's examine the Eden environment to see what we can discover.

SIGHT SENSE: A PLACE OF PEACE

Scenes of God's handiwork surrounded Adam and Eve in Eden: awesome oaks, fragrant flowers, lush shrubs, babbling brooks, majestic mountains, and peaceful ponds. And in all of God's work, order and simplicity prevailed.

Take a critical look at your personal environment. Is simplicity and order the rule or the exception? After a routine cleaning of your home, does it still feel cluttered? Stacks of old magazines scattered about? Closets stuffed with clothes you rarely or never wear? Too many appliances crowding your kitchen counter space? Whether we realize it or not, the very sight of clutter saps our energy, drains our strength, and depletes our sense of peace.

As curious as it may sound, many people have found that by uncluttering their environment they begin to free their thoughts, their emotions, and even their priorities. A simple, clean environment helps to clear your mind and create a greater sense of peace.

To establish a sense of visual warmth in your home, display objects that awaken good memories. Surround yourself with things that bring a feeling of peace, comfort, and joy. Perhaps your treasures are pictures of family and friends—or awards or honors that you've earned and received. Art may bring you energy: paintings full of color, sculptures brimming with life. Display items that remind you to dream—that draw you to God.

Before his death Henri Matisse, the great modern French painter, spent many months bedridden with colon cancer. His family moved his bed so he could take in the view of the countryside from the bedroom window. More important, they kept changing what was on his windowsill—so he could be continually inspired to paint. He did some of his most famous pieces from his bed.

Why not take a cue from the Matisse family? Add a little visual spice to your space. Try rotating or alternating your family photos, artwork, and displays. Many picture frames now hold several pictures at once, so you can change the subjects often. You can also treat them as a traveling art show by shifting them from room to room. A change of location also works well with plants. Besides being aesthetically pleasing, the visual variety may inspire you to new levels of personal creativity—as it did for Henri Matisse.

Another way to add visual zest to your personal space is to let the sunshine in. Open the blinds, draw back the curtain, thrown open the shutters, and let the natural light pour in. Sunlight has many benefits—among them the ability to cheer you by brightening your personal space. A lighter home is often a brighter home.

In their book *Health Power: Health by Choice, Not Chance,* Aileen Ludington and Hans Diehl suggest that sunlight has a lot to offer. In proper amounts it enhances the immune system, alleviates pain from swollen arthritic joints, relieves certain premenstrual symptoms, and lowers blood cholesterol levels. Sunlight can lift your spirits, improve your sleep, and increase your energy. Consult your doctor or dermatologist about how to enjoy the benefits of sunlight safely.

As you strive to make your personal environment a little piece of paradise, pay attention to the visuals that surround you. Clear away the clutter and move toward simplicity. You'll find that the loss is really a gain.

SMELL SENSE: MAKING GOOD SCENTS

Smell has become big business. From supermarkets and drugstores to department stores and boutiques, everyone seems to be getting into the trade of selling good scents. But which is the right scent for you?

A good place to start is to head back to the garden. What did God do to enhance the sense of smell in Eden? For one thing, He filled it with plants—all sorts of plants. Considering that more than 55,000 species of flowering plants grow in the Amazon rain forest, just imagine what Eden must have been like. Flowering and nonflowering plants. Leafy plants and creeping plants. Water plants and land plants. Such enormous variety. Of course they were beautiful to look at, but they also cleaned the air.

> *"Smell is a potent wizard that transports us across thousands of miles and all the years we have lived."*
> —*Helen Keller*

So take a tip from the Creator and place plenty of plants in your personal space. When you do, you'll be increasing the quality of the air you breathe (scientific research from NASA has shown that foliage and flowering plants have the ability to purify the air). Sure, it takes a little work, but the rewards are great.

Beyond flowers and plants, try other creative methods to make your space more fragrant. One way is to light the scented candles you find available in specialty shops, grocery stores, department stores, and pharmacies. Here are just a few of the many scents available—and what they can do for you:

Eucalyptus clears the head and invigorates the mind.

Chamomile is said to bring relaxation.

Pine is thought to stimulate creativity.

Orange is supposed to refresh the mind.

Tea Tree is said to ground your thoughts.

Thyme is believed to refresh and strengthen the immune system.

Cucumber is thought to calm the nerves.

Find a few scents that you enjoy, and bring them home to try. You'll be wonderfully pleased with the tranquil frame of mind they help create.

Still other ways exist to freshen the scent of your environment: aromatherapy kits, potpourri pots, air freshener plug-ins, room sprays, car deodorizing trees, bubble baths, body lotions, and scented oils. And don't forget about the perfume or cologne you wear. They are a great way to show your good scents.

Discover what fragrances are your favorites—and surround yourself with them.

SOUND SENSE:
TUNE IN TO LIFE'S NATURAL RHYTHMS

A day spent in nature is a day surrounded by sound. The playful rustle of wind dancing through trees. The soothing coos of a mourning dove. The ceaseless rhythm of the ocean. The enchanting chirp of crickets on a summer's eve. Swirling water tumbling over itself in a lively brook. The peaceful patter of rain on leafy trees. Thunder rumbling across the sky. Nature is a veritable symphony of sound. And God is its great conductor.

Back in the garden, Adam and Eve became accustomed to living by the natural rhythms of life.

They had no clocks, so they rose with the sun and slept with the stars—the natural rhythm of a day.

They worked six days and rested on the seventh—the natural rhythm of a week.

They grew and gathered food—the natural rhythm of seasons.

They had no radio or CD players, so their music was the melody of nature—the natural rhythm of sound.

In contrast to the soothing sounds of Eden, the average office today is likely to be filled with the constant drone of ringing phones, beeping pagers, and whining fax machines. And out of the office you and I will encounter honking traffic, blaring radios, noisy malls, and endlessly chattering televisions. The constant clamor can make it difficult to clear our minds and think.

"In twentieth-century society," comments Steven Halpern, contemporary musician, "the noise level is such that it keeps knocking our bodies out of tune and out of their natural rhythms. This ever-increasing assault of sound upon our ears, minds, and bodies adds to the stress load of civilized beings trying to live in a highly complex environment."

Artist Luigi Russolo observed that "in antiquity there was only silence. In the nineteenth century, with the invention of the machine, noise was born. Today, noise triumphs and reigns supreme."

The Garden of Eden, a place of perfect peace, stands in striking contrast to the modern world of manufactured noise. What can we do to save our sanity? Let's explore three possible alternatives to the increasing assault of sound on our personal environments.

✓ **Silence.** In a noisy, clamoring, overstimulated society, silence seems like a lost art. Indeed, many have become so accustomed to noise that they actually feel uncomfortable in silence. Some even prefer to fall asleep at night with the television or radio on. British poet Dame Edith Sitwell once remarked, "My personal hobbies are reading, listening to music, and silence." Sometimes the best thing you can do is to shut out sound of every kind and sit in silence. Somewhere in the silence you may find it easier to tune in to God's voice as He speaks to you of His love.

✓ **Natural rhythms.** To restore a sense of peace and harmony to your home (or workplace), consider filling it with sounds from nature—the natural rhythms designed by the Creator to bring rest to the spirit. You might start by looking into nature CDs. Many companies offer high-quality recordings of nature for your enjoyment: ocean waves, gurgling brooks, gentle rain, waterfalls, wind through the trees, birds in song, and the many voices of the rain forest. Some artists have set these soothing sounds to relaxing instrumental music. Find out which ones help you to relax.

Inexpensive sound generators are also widely available today. They generate natural sounds to help drown out unwanted background noise. If you happen to live in a noisy city or next to a heavily trafficked road, you might find a sound generator useful. They can often reproduce the rhythms of rain, waterfalls, rivers, and the beating of ocean surf. If you're a pet lover, you may want to consider owning a songbird. Another restful sound is that of a tabletop fountain—and of course fountains are also enjoyable to watch.

✓ **Relaxing music.** Music, it's been said, is simply noise that someone has organized. Many studies suggest that music has a calming effect on the human body and mind. Listening to soothing music may reduce stress, decrease muscle tension, strengthen the immune system, raise endorphin levels, and produce feelings of peace. No one kind of music soothes and relaxes everyone. Many enjoy the piano, flute, guitar, or harp. Others prefer classical music or smooth jazz. Discover the style that makes you feel relaxed and at peace. Then keep it handy when stress starts to rise.

TASTE SENSE:
TANTALIZE YOUR TASTE BUDS NATURALLY

When it came to food in the Garden of Eden,

Adam and Eve ate like the king and queen they were, for the God who made them provided what was best for them. Everything they needed for perfect health was right there in the garden.

Genesis 1:29 gives us the basic description: "Then God said, 'I give you every seed-bearing plant on the face of the whole earth and every tree that has fruit with seed in it. They will be yours for food.'" It was a simple yet wonderful menu.

The original human diet as designed by God Himself was to be a vegetarian one consisting of fruits and vegetables, grains and nuts. And every bite was to be a delight. Adam and Eve had the most delicious berries, the ripest apples, the juiciest oranges, the plumpest plums, the tastiest nuts, the freshest grains, the yellowest squash, the best potatoes, the sweetest tomatoes, and the crunchiest cucumbers. In addition, they had the purest water for refreshment. It was all theirs for the choosing.

> *"And God, thank You for the peas."*
> —*Four-year-old Mark*

Tasting the treasures of nature is one of God's greatest gifts. Eating may be a necessity, but enjoying the experience is not. Yet God in His goodness gave us pleasure in food. Of course, some food choices are better than others. And our modern track record has not been so good.

Often we substitute sugary snacks for the sweetness of fruit. We trade the goodness of vegetables for fast fatty foods. Many of us swap the vitality of pure water for sweetened syrupy drinks. As a result we exchange healthy nutrition for empty calories. The result is taste buds that become accustomed to the assault of sugars, fats, and nutrition-free foods. It's no wonder that we find little pleasure in God's natural eating plans.

Even when we do try to eat a healthy diet, too many of us don't take the time to enjoy it. Busy people with hectic lives grab a meal on the run—one hand on our food, the other on our work. Or we eat while being entertained, diminishing the actual meal experience.

Would you like to try an experiment? Tonight for dinner, actually sit at a table while not allowing any outside distractions: no TV, no phone, no newspaper, no mail, no work assignments. Take the time to really look at your food. Notice all the colors and textures. Listen as you eat for the sounds that it creates. Relish the texture of the food in your mouth. Savor the smells. Take in the tastes. Don't rush through the meal with your thoughts on what you have to do next. God gave you the sense of taste to enhance your life. Enjoy it!

Let every bite be a delight.

TOUCH SENSE:
THRIVING THROUGH THE GENTLE TOUCH

Would an all-powerful God ever create something that was incomplete? unfinished? not whole? Apparently so. Seems rather hard to believe, but in the midst of perfection something was found lacking—like a bare patch of canvas on an artist's finished masterpiece. But there it was—God's unfinished business.

In the Genesis account of Creation God made the earth in just seven days. At the end of each day He stood back to examine His handiwork. For five days in a row His assessment was the same: "And God saw that it was good." But on the sixth day something unusual occurred. For the first time He said that part of Creation was "not good." Here's the exact quote from Genesis 2:18: "The Lord God said, 'It is not good for the man to be alone. I will make a helper suitable for him.'"

After His wondrous work in creating Adam, the first man, God said that something was amiss. The human being needed a partner. A life mate. A love mate. Someone to hold his hand as he walked through the garden. Someone to slip his arm around as the sun sank into the west. Someone to snuggle with as the stars came out. Someone to have and to hold for a lifetime. And so God created Eve. She was Adam's equal in every way. Together they were to rule the world—in love with God and in love with each other.

What was true at Creation is still so today—people need others to survive and thrive. We each require helpmates and heart mates to make it through life. One of the ways we can aid each other to flourish is through the wonderful gift of touch. The skin God created for each of us is the largest sense organ in our bodies and responds positively to every loving touch. Numerous studies document the fact that we must have touch to develop and grow. Research has shown that husbands who hug their wives regularly tend to live longer and have fewer heart problems. In his book *Psychosocial Medicine: A Study of the Sick Society*

James L. Halliday writes that infants deprived of regular maternal body contact can develop profound depression with an accompanying lack of appetite and wasting so severe that it can lead to death.

> *"'Lord, if you are willing, you can make me whole.'*
> *Jesus reached out and touched the man. 'I am*
> *willing,' he said. 'Be clean.'"*
> *—Matthew 8:2, 3*
> *(describing the healing of a leper)*

Somewhere deep in the fabric of the human heart God placed a desire to love and be loved. Touch and be touched. Well-known family therapist Virginia Satir once stated that we need four hugs a day for survival, eight a day for maintenance, and 12 a day for growth. How do you express your need for human contact? Do you have someone you can turn to for a soothing word and a gentle touch? If not, one of the best ways to find such a friend is to be that kind of friend to others.

We can also enjoy our God-given sense of touch through the textures around us. Velvety pillows and rough burlap. Silky clothes and coarse carpeting. Smooth grass and sharp stones. All are sensations we experience through the sense of touch. In your personal environment have you taken the time to surround yourself with things you like to feel?

Are there feathery pillows to caress your head as you snuggle into bed? Do you have a favorite overstuffed chair you can flop into and relax? Is your home carpeting gentle on the feet? Do you wear comfortable clothing that's soft on the skin? The next time you go shopping, try a different approach. Rather than simply searching for the latest styles, try *feeling* the fabric first. Run your hand down the clothing rack or over the shelves until you find something pleasant to the touch. Only then should you pull it out and take a look at the style. If you need extra guidance, ask a sales attendant for help in finding natural fiber fabric. The softer texture is sure to be a sensation explosion next to your skin. You might be surprised how much better you feel in clothing chosen for comfort rather than chic.

Take some time this week to explore creative ways you can make your personal environment a more touching place to be.

WHEN YOU CAN'T CHANGE THINGS . . .

Especially in the workplace you may struggle with limitations on how much you can alter your environment. Not everyone wants your "soothing music" floating into their ears—not to mention your pet songbird. When you can't quite attain Edenlike beauty on the outside, try doing it within.

A few years ago a hospital nurse was getting frustrated with an old copy machine that produced copies very very slowly. On one particular occasion, while waiting for her job to finish, she decided she wasn't going to let it frustrate her—she would use that time to pray. She made a particular request to the Lord—and her prayer received an answer. The next time she made copies, she prayed again. And again. "Over a period of time," she said, "I found myself in front of that machine, taking more and more requests to the Lord." And she kept getting positive responses.

When she shared her experience with some of her fellow workers, they started doing the same thing. It got to the point where they began keeping a list of the requests and the date on which the Lord had answered the prayer. Soon they went from despising that old copy machine to treasuring it.

So even if it seems you can't change your environment for the better, you really can.

"Do not be conformed to this world, but be transformed by the renewing of your mind, that you may prove what is that good and acceptable and perfect will of God" (Romans 12:2, NKJV).

LIFESTYLE CHANGES YOU CAN BEGIN TODAY

You don't have to visit every national park or spend days watching the Discovery Channel to enjoy the environment. God's Creation is all around you. Choose to notice, and enjoy it!

1. Sight—Add beautiful sights to your personal world. Place a plant on your office desk. Add a bouquet of flowers to the kitchen table. Hang a calendar or other photographs of nature on a wall you look at often. Buy a low-maintenance Beta fish and make friends with it.

2. Sound—Change the sounds you hear by adding peaceful music to your life. *Really listen* to the music, don't just use it as background noise. Close your eyes to keep out distractions. Try Pachabel's *Canon in D*, Hayden's *Cello Concerto in C*, or Debussey's

Claire de Lune. Choose one of the *Songs of Health and Healing* CDs from Integrity Music and play it in your office.

3. Touch—Use touch everyday to lead a happier, more aware life. Reach out for a friend's arm when engaged in conversation. Ask for and give appropriate hugs. Notice the physical sensation of your clothes—cotton, rayon, silk, wool, etc.

4. Taste—Be adventurous! Eat a variety of colors—yellow, orange, brown, red, and green. (Chocolate, by the way, counts as brown!) Choose crunchy whole-grain breads and cereals to wake up your taste buds. Use moderate amounts of sugar, salt, and fats. Revel in new flavors.

5. Smell—Even smell can help you be healthier. Burn a scented candle (in a safe place). Fill a bowl with potpourri and put it in the living room. Have a fragrant bouquet of flowers on your bedside table. Inhale deeply the scent of a rose. Revel in the fragrances God has placed near you.

Your environment influences your health. As often as you can, establish one that fosters peace and well-being. Remember the importance of fresh air and sunlight. Try to have a home situation that allows you to relax. Remember the benefits of sight and aromatherapy. Enjoy both music and silence. Choose to take time with your meals. And never forget the wonderfully healthy benefit of hugging and embracing those you love.

5

The Real
Fountain of Youth

The "A" in CREATION Health stands for *Activity*. Activity means finding every muscle you can and using it! God made all of those muscles for a reason and designed us so that activity is key to living God's prescription for full life. Active people are more alert, energetic, fun, caring, and alive!

Activity strengthens the body to fight disease. In fact, purposeful activity may be the best medicine for fighting almost any disease. It helps the body battle stress, anxiety, and depression. It enables you to sleep better, look better, and feel better. It's all part of God's plan to fill your daily adventure with joy, peace, hope, love, patience, kindness, and good health.

So go ahead and get active. The benefits of a healthier life await you!

SCIENTIFIC SUPPORT FOR *ACTIVITY*

The verdict is in. Research during the past few decades has clearly shown that physical activity can reduce the incidence of colon cancer in men and breast cancer in women. The only question is how? Some studies suggest that exercise results in the production of immune system-modulating chemicals called cytokines. Or it may reduce colon exposure to potential carcinogens by speeding gut peristalsis (the rate the intestines move waste products through the body). Other researchers have suggested that it reduces estrogen-modulating fat. But it doesn't really matter how it works. Regular exercise lowers the risk of cancer. That is reason enough to be active.

HIV is no longer an automatic death sentence, especially for people who engage in moderate exercise. Physical activity has been shown to enhance the quality of life as well as survival in those with the disease. Moderate exercise also enhances several measures of immunity in infected patients. Be careful, though, because more is not necessarily better when applied to exercise. Intense activity may temporarily suppress the immune system.

Glutamine is an amino acid essential for normal functioning of the immune system as well as many other body processes. However, the main source in humans is skeletal muscle. Research has revealed that either too much or insufficient exercise can impair health. That's thought to be one of the reasons why both marathon runners and sedentary individuals are more susceptible to upper respiratory infections. A proven link exists between skeletal muscle and immunity. It is best activated through physical activity—exercise.

THE *REAL* FOUNTAIN OF YOUTH

In 1493 Spanish explorer Juan Ponce de León stepped aboard a ship bound for America. He would share the voyage with famed explorer Christopher Columbus, who was on his second journey to the

New World. Ponce de León didn't embark on the expedition as a sightseeing trip, however. He set sail with one goal, one vision, one desire in mind: to find the legendary fountain of youth—that mythical spring of water that would grant eternal youth to the one who drank from it.

De León had many amazing adventures in the New World. History credits him as the first European to discover Florida. Conquering Puerto Rico, he eventually became its governor. But for all his long years of searching, he never discovered what his heart desired most—the source of perpetual youth.

Hundreds of years later people still continue Ponce de León's quest. Rather than searching for the fountain of youth in some undiscovered land, however, many today seek youthful vitality in pills, therapies, and special diets.

Is there a *real* source of eternal youth in this world? Not that we know of. But many researchers believe they have found the closest resource we have for fulfilling the promises of the legendary fountain of youth. It is simply physical activity.

"I'm trying to build strength. And that doesn't happen until the muscle fiber ruptures and the nerve fiber registers the pain. Then nature overcompensates and within 48 hours, the fiber is made stronger."
—Stephen R. Covey

When physically challenged through regular exercise, the human body grows stronger and healthier and ages more slowly. In fact, according to the American

Heart Association, regular activity has many whole-person health benefits, including great gains for the mind, body, spirit, and even social relationships.

Research has clearly shown that with regular physical activity the body sleeps better and is less susceptible to injury. Mentally, the body handles stress more effectively, the mind is able to think more clearly, and a person generally has a more positive outlook on life. Socially, people often gain more confidence because they feel and look better. And spiritually, those who exercise often find a deeper connection to their Creator, who made them for a life of health, happiness, and peace.

Sadly, the U.S. Preventive Services Task Force has stated that more than 70 percent of the population in the United States is not physically active. In fact, inactivity is said to be one of the greatest public health challenges of this century. Recent findings suggest that the incidence of stroke and Type II diabetes would be lower, high blood pressure could be prevented or reduced, and bone fractures would occur less often if America just *moved* more. That's why physicians such as James Rippe at Celebration Health emphasize exercise with their patients.

"We talk about physical activity with every single one of our clients," Rippe explains. "It's one of the pillars, one of the key things that we think is very important to good health. And I can tell you that when I see many of my patients a year later, they say, 'I have never felt better in my life.' Of course, as a physician, I know that they've also done something very good for their heart. We don't have any magic bullets in medicine, but the nearest to one is physical activity."

Rippe states that people who are physically active cut their risk of heart disease in half. On the flip side, that means that a person who is physically *inactive* has chosen the same level of increased risk as smoking a pack of cigarettes a day.

EDEN'S ACTIVITY

Activity is an important part of the CREATION model of health and a vital component of wholeness. And again this principle goes right back to the Garden of Eden.

The original paradise was indeed a beautiful, tranquil place. But contrary to some stereotypes, Adam and Eve didn't lie all day on a riverbank in Eden, drinking fresh coconut juice. They didn't just lounge around looking at flowers and birds. While the Creator *could* have designed their lives to be quite labor-free and passive, He had something else in mind.

"The Lord God took the man and put him in the Garden of Eden to work it and take care of it" (Genesis 2:15). Paradise, for Adam and Eve, wasn't a world of idleness. Eden didn't automatically meet all their needs. They were responsible for cultivating the garden. It was God's way of keeping them physically active.

Studies done by Steven Blair at the Cooper Institute for Aerobics Research and by other groups have revealed the enormous influence of exercise on our daily lives. Simply getting up off the couch and walking for 30 to 40 minutes three to five times a week can diminish our risk of premature death from cancer and cardiovascular disease by 20 to 40 percent.

If I told you that I could give you a 20 to 40 percent return on an investment, you'd probably write me out a check right now.

"Exercise," explains physical therapist Terry Barter, "is the component that brings in the nutrients via the bloodstream to your muscles, your bones, and your joints. It helps get the oxygen through your blood system. This helps grow, mend, promote, and maintain your body. When you take in your car for a tune-up, it really runs better. Then after a while, it needs another tune-up. The body is the same way. Activity is the way we tune up."

EXERCISE AND THE MIND

Amazing as it might seem, physical exercise affects more than just our bodies. It also helps our minds.

Our bodily organs are intricately interrelated. Everything inside us influences everything else. The state of our lungs determines the condition of our hearts. Our stomachs affect our intestines. Beyond that, our bodies can sway our minds. Perhaps you've heard about how our mental outlook or our level of stress can impact our physical health. Well, that's a two-way street. Mind affects body. But body also affects mind. And regular exercise can improve the overall attitude of our minds. In fact, exercise has a variety of psychological effects that enhance physical health. It buffers against stress, is an effective treatment for anxiety, and according to some researchers, is as effective as psychotherapy in treating mild depression.

"In the past 20 years," James Rippe reports, "a tremendous and growing body of information suggests that mind and body are inextricably linked to each other. And I'm now seeing a number of people coming back a year or two after their first evaluation, and those people who have become more physically active tell me they have never felt better in their lives."

LIFE-CHANGE STORIES

Listen to the stories of two people for whom increased physical activity has made all the difference:

Jim Baez, director of purchasing, age 59; activity of choice: walking

"One year ago I was feeling pretty sick. Some examinations revealed that I had diabetes. I needed to make some changes in the way I took care of myself, otherwise I would increase the likelihood that I would have further complications.

"I started attending education classes on diabetes that brought me up to speed with what I had to do to change my eating habits. I learned how a good exercise routine and weight loss program could make dramatic improvements in my particular health situation. So I decided to start walking.

"When I began, I had to go pretty slowly, because I couldn't tolerate more than a mile at a time. But through the summer I kept at it, gradually building up stamina. Now I walk five miles every morning before I go into work. I've dropped 45 pounds off my weight, and during my latest visit with my doctor he officially took me off medication altogether. The exercise program had kept my blood glucose at the same levels it was when I was on medication. I've been able to get my life and health back under control.

"The best result, I think, is that I feel so much better than I did a year ago. I'm healthier. The walk in the morning takes about one hour and 15 minutes. It gives me time to reflect and get my mind prepared for the day ahead. In addition to the physical benefits of exercising, it's helped me to organize my thoughts and think things through in a way that I didn't have the time to do before I began walking. If I don't have thoughts that need sorting, it's a wonderful time for quiet meditation.

"I wish you could talk to my wife about the changes in me. She says I'm a totally different person. My attitude is more positive, and I'm less prone to be short-tempered. She's happy that I've gotten this thing under control.

"The best tip I could give you is: *persevere*. Don't give up. You'll need to assume a tremendous amount of discipline to get it done. But while changing life habits takes a lot of work and commitment, it's worth it.

Wendy Sullivan, office manager, age 30; activities of choice: walking, running

"I never had to watch my weight until after the birth of my second child. Those 10 extra pounds wouldn't go away, and my weight continued going up from there. One day I woke up, looked at myself, and said, 'I can't live like this anymore. I have to do something about it.'

"I started an active exercise program about a year ago as a New Year's resolution. Since then I've lost 24 pounds. Actually, I lost the weight in the first six months of training, and for the past six months I've held steady. For a while I tried to lose just a bit more, but I've stopped. My body seems to be telling me this is the right weight for me.

"At first I started out with a simple exercise program, walking regularly, then working my way up to running. Since then I've participated in two small races—each of them five kilometers. Before I started the program I was drinking six to eight Cokes per day, but I quickly cut those out. Caffeine withdrawal gave me tremendous headaches, and I became grumpy. But that time quickly passed, and I had no further problems. Now I drink mainly water.

"Not only do I feel better physically, but I also perform better mentally—partly because I know that I look better. It's nice to hear people say, 'Wow, I didn't even recognize you. You look great!' That gives me more satisfaction than anything, and it really cheers me.

"My routine has affected my family. As soon as I started my weight-loss program, my mother did the same thing. She's now dropped about 60 pounds, and it's made such a difference. So my husband decided to get into the spirit. He started exercising with us, and he's taken off 35 pounds. It's really nice to do a program with someone else. We can compare weights and encourage each other.

"If someone were to ask my advice about starting an activity program, I would tell them to realize that it is a lifestyle change. I thought there was no way I could lose 15 pounds. But I tell you, when that first five pounds dropped, I thought, *Wow, this is so great!*

Then I had a real goal: if I could lose five, I could go all the way. You don't have to be obsessive about weight loss. Just live a healthy lifestyle and let your body find its natural weight."

ADVICE FROM THREE PROFESSIONALS
Jeannine Chobotar, Physical Therapist

"When someone comes to a physical therapist for help, we usually focus our efforts on three areas: *strength, endurance,* and *flexibility*. These are the three key components of a physically sound body. Many people forget that it is important to focus on improving the condition of the whole body, not just one particular area. We often begin by establishing an exercise program that concentrates on strength training.

"One of the major health problems people face today in our country is inactivity. When people are inactive or have very low levels of activity, their muscles begin to atrophy. That means they get smaller and weaker.

"A hundred years ago people got most of the exercise they needed just by doing their chores and other daily activities. It kept them strong enough that they didn't need health clubs, stationary bikes, or exercise programs to stay healthy. Today, however, with our sedentary lifestyles, we have to make a conscious, consistent effort to exercise and stay healthy so our muscles don't grow small and weak.

"Because our bodies are living, changing organisms, it is really impossible for us to stay at a constant level of health physically, so we must strengthen our body by challenging it, pushing it bit by bit. Some people deceive themselves by thinking that if they just eat healthfully they will have good health. While a good diet is important, it's not enough. If you're not challenging your body, you're not strengthening it, and all the functions of your body start declining.

"Another problem with inactivity is that inactive muscles become stiff and more open to injury. That makes flexibility a crucial part of physical conditioning. When you are active and challenging your muscles, a stretching process takes place that adds flexibility and strength, making injury less likely.

"When I work with patients, I try to emphasize the importance of being active every day, not just two or three times a week. I usually give them 'homework,' exercises they can to do at home. As we get closer to the end of our treatments, I encourage them to maintain their exercise in any way that motivates them. As soon as people stop exercising they start getting weaker again, so it's very important to remain active.

"Endurance, built up by aerobic and cardiovascular training, is also a vital component of physical health. Such exercises work the heart and lungs, causing them to become stronger and more efficient. Endurance exercise elevates the heart rate for a sustained period of time and gives you more energy throughout the day. This type of exercise is especially important for people who spend most of their day on a job that doesn't require much physical exertion. When you train your heart through endurance training, you will have more energy!

"Strength training, flexibility training, and endurance training. Be sure to include all of them in your exercise plan. You will feel less tired, you will feel more motivated, and you will have a greater joy for life in general. Activity makes you feel good!"

Brenda Duerksen, Registered Nurse and Health Educator

"When a patient first comes into my office and clearly is not living at an optimum level of health, I usually begin by asking them what kind of exercise they get. Unfortunately, the typical answer is 'I do not exercise at all.'

"Many patients I see get so little exercise that they have a hard time just doing the day-to-day things. They are in such poor physical shape that just the effort it takes to move around is extremely tiring.

"When I think about the importance of activity, several of the patients I work with come to mind. One of them is a little woman in her 70s who has diabetes Type II, which means she's not on insulin but taking the anti-diabetic medication. She was having a difficult time keeping her blood sugar levels in the proper range. I challenged her to start a regular walking program, exercising every day, if possible. She did, and brought her blood sugar levels down about 30 points in three months while also losing five or six pounds. When she came back for a follow-up visit she was glowing. Sold on walking, she is determined to make these changes stick for the rest of her life.

"Anyone can exercise. If you are homebound, there are all sorts of interesting exercises that can be done in the home just for the legs. If you can get to a shopping mall, most malls have daily walking programs in which you can stroll with others in safety before the stores open.

"The most difficult part to adopting a more active, healthy lifestyle is not picking what kind of exercise to do, where to do it, or how often to do it. It is actually *doing it!*

"We urge three helpful tools for our patients:

"1. Find an exercise partner. If you have a buddy you have to meet at the corner or who is going to stop by and pick you up, it is a great motivator.

"2. List the benefits. When you write down the anticipated benefits, you are more likely to stick with an exercise activity. Think about losing weight, breathing better, sleeping more soundly, avoiding headaches, not feeling so fatigued, and finding new joy with your friends and family.

"3. Consider the alternatives. Sometimes the scare tactic is the best motivation.

"Recent studies have shown an ever-increasing problem with childhood obesity. Some reports indicate that the number of overweight children is doubling every 10 to 20 years. Unfortunately, children learn from adults. They watch us, and learn it is OK to sit in front of a television or computer for hours and hours and hours. Less and less often we see children outside running around the yard, jumping rope, climbing trees, riding bikes, and swimming. But these are normal things children like to do, activities that will help them enjoy God's prescription for health.

"One of the best things for a healthy family to do together is to participate in more physical activities.

Plan events that get you into the outdoors doing active things you find enjoyable. Activities shared together are rewarding, both in terms of growing relationships and increased health."

Rhonda Ringer, M.D., Family Practice Physician

"In my primary care practice I've found that there is almost no patient who cannot benefit by increased physical activity. In fact, I believe such activity may be the best medicine there is for practically any health problem because it strengthens the body to fight disease. I think people grasp this principle instinctively because they usually tell me, 'Oh yeah, I know I need to exercise more.'

"The reason so many don't exercise isn't really a lack of awareness; the problem is busy schedules that lead to overloaded lifestyles. Once we abandon exercise, everything starts to flop out of kilter. Weight goes up, we do not sleep as well, anxiety increases, sugar gets out of control, blood pressure creeps up, and cholesterol rises.

"But none of that needs to happen. Exercise makes a difference! In my experience, people uniformly feel better and sleep better when they exercise. That's *100 percent of the time!*

"When active people have fallen out of practice, I remind them about how good they felt and the results they achieved when they were active. If those memories can be restimulated in their brain, they are much more likely to say, 'Yeah, I need to start doing that again, because I felt so much better then.' Some remember how their blood sugar stayed under control or their blood pressure lowered. Others recall how they gained 10 pounds in three months when they stopped exercising. If I can reconnect them to the positive things they remember from when they were active, it's much easier for them to get back into it again.

"If people have never been very active, or they tell me they hate exercise, that's much more difficult. I may start by reminding them of some of the benefits they will reap from getting active. We're not discussing the Olympics here—we're talking about starting out just 10 minutes a day. Most people tell me that they can do 10 minutes a day. Then I ask them if they can do it every day. If not, I get them to do it as many days a week as they can. *Ten minutes a day can help you feel 100 percent better!*

"Occasionally someone will ask me what my favorite exercises are for staying healthy. That's easy. My favorite exercises are just that—doing whatever I enjoy most.

"Whatever physical activity that you can do and enjoy doing is what you should do. For example, if an older individual tells me that they love to pull weeds in their garden or work in their yard for 15 minutes at a time, I say, 'Super duper.' I recommend what is easiest and most economical, because that is what is going to be incorporated with the best success.

"When we talk about exercise, we often discuss it in terms of its benefits to such conditions as diabetes, hypertension, cholesterol, and heart disease. Three of the best results of consistent exercise are stress release, depression release, and insomnia release. Though we don't talk about it much, increased activity can significantly improve all these conditions, because it raises the level of the endorphins in our body that are the body's own 'uppers.' Activity dissipates the epinephrine, and norepinephrine the stress hormones. It drops the cortisol, an immune system depressor. A number of studies show that a program of activity over a period of several weeks is as effective as a prescription antidepressant for depression treatment.

"I believe it is more difficult to listen to what God is whispering into our souls when we are overstimulated. If we can exercise while enjoying nature, it can be a time when we really come together mentally, emotionally, and spiritually. Such activity helps us to calm down, quiet the spirit, and silence the clamor in our brain. Exercise provides time to decide where we're headed and what choices are best. It allows us time to examine what God thinks and what He wants us to do versus what society or our employer is demanding that we do. All of us need to have quiet time to stop and process.

"By the way, exercise can also improve our relationships. Take a revitalizing walk in the evening or a refreshing walk in the morning with someone you love. Couples who do tell me it is one of the best times they have for sharing together. It's an opportunity for coming together, of cherishing each other without a lot of distractions.

"The act of exercising is an antidepressant, encouraging, strengthening, feel-good-about-yourself medication in and of itself. It puts you in a frame of mind to enable you to relate more positively to people around you. No pill can do that as well as muscle movement, especially when it is done outdoors regularly with friends!"

Lifestyle Changes You Can Begin Today

Whatever our individual tastes and limitations, the Creator has designed us for meaningful activity. It should always be a part of our lives.

Keep these suggestions in mind:

- ✓ Always see your doctor before starting any exercise program.
- ✓ Your exercise should be something that you enjoy doing. The more pleasure it gives you, the more you will do it.
- ✓ Almost everyone can benefit by increased physical activity. In fact, it may be the best medicine there is for practically any disease.
- ✓ Start slowly but have definite measurable goals. Ideally you should work your way up to at least 30 minutes of activity three times a week.
- ✓ If possible, have an exercise companion.
- ✓ Exercise is a great antidepressant. The next time you're feeling down, go outside for a brisk walk.
- ✓ An exercise program can improve your relationships by helping you to look and feel better.

Start walking—for yourself and for those you love!

6

How Faith
Affects Your Health

The "T" in CREATION Health stands for *Trust in Divine Power*. The Creator designed us to be His friends. But sometimes our lives seem so busy that we leave little time for Him. Those are the times we try to go it alone, without the wisdom and energy His friendship offers. Yet without Him, our daily activities become rather colorless, like paintings by an artist who has no heart.

Alone I'm a little frightened. With Him, I'm eager to face the world!

SCIENTIFIC SUPPORT FOR *TRUST IN DIVINE POWER*

A study of 560 households has revealed that people who pray are happier, more satisfied, and enjoy a deeper sense of well-being about the direction their lives are headed. In addition, those with religious allegiance are significantly less likely to experience physical illness, mental symptoms, or difficulties with socialization. Researchers have offered many explanations. They range from adherence to the healthy lifestyle prescribed by religious teachings to divine intervention. Future studies will be required to identify the reason why trust in a divine power is a pathway to optimal physical and mental health. In the meantime, the scientific data clearly indicates that opening your heart to God will enrich you in ways other than through improved spiritual health.

Depression is both a symptom and a syndrome. It can be triggered by a major upheaval in your life and can, by itself, cause major changes in your health. Scientists have shown that depression can worsen the symptoms of pain, result in greater reporting of physical illness symptoms, and lessen the likelihood that its victims will engage in healthy pursuits. No wonder trust in a divine power has the potential to influence so many aspects of mental and physical health. That's because religion has proven to be a highly effective means by which to reduce depression. This is especially true of those with conservative theological beliefs and those with large amounts of social support.

A study of 855 high school seniors revealed that students who go to church are less likely to become delinquents, drink alcohol, or use marijuana than other adolescents—an observation that applied to both boys and girls. Clearly, there is an important role for religious commitment and moral education in maintaining a healthy society.

HOW FAITH AFFECTS YOUR HEALTH

Disease squashed in the face of trust? Chronic illness bowing out before faith? It may seem unrealistic, but recent studies are beginning to unveil the connection between religion and recovery.

A May 2001 *Reader's Digest* article, "Why Doctors Now Believe Faith Heals," cited several studies done by such reputable institutions as Duke University and Dartmouth Medical School that link personal belief and personal health. Among the findings:

- ✓ Those who attended religious services more than once a week enjoyed a seven-year-longer life expectancy than those who never attended.
- ✓ Older adults who considered themselves religious functioned better and had fewer problems than the nonreligious.
- ✓ Patients comforted by their faith were three times more likely to be living six months after open-heart surgery than those who found no emotional support in religion.
- ✓ Among the 400 Caucasian men studied in Evans County, Georgia, those who considered religion very important and who attended church regularly had a significant protective effect against high blood pressure
- ✓ Adults who attend a house of worship have lower rates of depression and anxiety.

"I fully believe," says Ted Hamilton, of Florida Hospital, "and there is research that's beginning to support the notion, that trust actually releases healing hormones into our bodies that contribute to the healing process. Now the research is not as definitive as we'd like for it to be, but my guess is that five years from now we will view trust and hope as medications to help people recover more quickly."

The scientific data is growing. Georgetown University Medical School professor Dale Matthews and his colleagues have shown that religious involvement helps people avoid illness, recover from it more quickly, and most remarkably, live longer. The more spiritually committed you are, the more you benefit. Medical internist Larry Dossey and others have published rather extensively on the benefits of prayer and healing. Undeniably, the medical community has a growing respect for the role that faith and prayer play in our overall well-being.

> *"Any concern too small to be turned into a prayer is too small to be made into a burden."*
> —Mille Thomton

"I found that people who are faced with disease," continues Hamilton, "who are also fearful about the ultimate outcome, have more difficulty focusing on recovery. But those who have, beneath all the concerns and worries and challenges of that illness, an underlying trust, a trust that says things will ultimately work out for the good because God loves and God cares for them—they're somehow able to marshal resources that contribute to their healing in ways that others aren't able to."

A HEALING FAITH

Faith is an essential part of healing as well as a vital aspect of wholeness. It can keep us strong even when physically we're at our weakest. And it can sustain us even when our bodies lose the battle for life. I believe a personal faith in Jesus Christ makes an eternal difference in daily healing.

Florida Hospital chaplain Dick Tibbits has found this to be true for many of the patients he counsels.

"Some people have to face the reality of a terminal illness or a crisis situation," he says, "and where do they turn? At such times faith and trust in God become extremely important, because faith in God gives strength that allows people to cope with such overwhelming news. In fact, sometimes after the death of a loved one, trust in God may be the only thing that helps people deal with the tragedy. It's the belief that He will take care of us, even after death, that allows people to be able to find the strength to cope."

A GROWING FAITH

The story of Creation illustrates the importance of trust in God. He designed everything in the Garden of Eden to inspire confidence in Him as someone who would care for humanity.

The Creator surrounded Adam and Eve with living things that were very good (see Genesis 1). He wanted them to know that He was the Great Provider, that they could count on Him to care for their needs. God wanted the first human couple to grow into a healthy relationship with Him.

But the Creation story can teach us something else about trust. It's evident that Adam and Eve had to *grow* in their confidence in God. Faith is a process, not just an on-and-off switch.

At first they stumbled in their relationship with Him. God had warned them about one spot in Eden where they should not go—the tree of the knowledge of good and evil. That's where a deceiver lay in wait. Holding a grudge against the Creator, he wanted to hurt God's children.

But Eve saw a delightful fruit hanging there. It looked good. What harm could there be in it? She listened to the serpent instead of the voice of the God who loved her—who had provided for her. Eve ignored divine instructions and ate the fruit. Then she convinced Adam to share it with her. And just that quickly both the man and the woman shattered their relationship of trust.

But afterward the Creator came looking for them. He sought to restore their broken relationship and rebuild that trust.

Our human parents needed to trust God even when their impulses led them in another direction. And Adam and Eve did learn to trust—the hard way.

You see, faith is a process. It is something we grow into—something we develop.

Now, you may be thinking that you don't have the kind of faith that produces miracles. That your faith is rather weak. Well, guess what? Jesus' disciples had the same concern. They were always encountering obstacles that seemed bigger than their faith.

So they came up to Him one day and said, "'Increase our faith.' So the Lord said, 'If you have faith as a mustard seed, you can say to this mulberry tree, "Be pulled up by the roots and be planted in the sea" and it would obey you'" (Luke 17:5, 6, NKJV).

A tiny seed of faith. That's all it takes. Why? Because what matters is *whom* we place our faith in. If we put it in an all-powerful Creator, then anything can happen, anything is possible. And it's not because our faith is so big—it's because of the size of our God.

The Bible tells us that this same God offered the ultimate gift to the world: His one and only Son. He sent His Son to rescue us from the disaster of sin. In the person of Jesus Christ, God the Father gave everything. Emptying heaven, He held nothing back—because we were in need.

Paul talks about this awesome generosity in one of his letters: "He who did not spare his own Son, but gave him up for us all—how will he not also, along with him, graciously give us all things?" (Romans 8:32).

Through His gift of the one closest to His heart He will provide us freely with all good things.

That's the God we can trust. We can have absolute confidence in Him in sickness and in health. And we can look to Him for healing and wholeness.

A CHANGING FAITH

"Trust changes a person's outlook," observes Florida Hospital chaplain Marti Jones. "Trusting people are more positive. When they know that God cares for them, they are able to rely on the fact that God is leading, even in the physical care they're receiving.

"One of the ministries that I carry on in the hospital," Jones continues, "is providing spiritual nurture not only for our patients, but also for our staff. We have a ministry called People of the Word—POW. Weekly we study the Bible with individuals who want to come together and explore it. That's how I met Barbara Oilelette."

Barbara Oilelette will never forget how studying the Bible helped her find trust and changed her entire life.

"The first time I met Marti," Barbara recalls, "I was at a really low time in my life. My husband of 35 years had left me. I was devastated. Then a few months later my healthy mom died suddenly. She had a massive stroke. I felt as if I had nothing left, so I turned to God.

"Because we're human," she acknowledges, "it's hard to trust people. But I found that if we trust God fully and hand Him all our cares, He gives us peace. He provides us the support and the love that we need.

"When your husband leaves you, you feel kind of worthless. Some people reach out to the bottle or to drugs. Others get on the phone and talk to their friends. But I felt full trust in the Lord, because He'll never leave me—and I knew that. I joined the Bible study that Marti was teaching, and since then I've grown closer to the Lord."

"I still complain that God is silent. But I am not as frightened of the silence as I once was. Silence is not taken for rejection anymore. Silence is just that, silence—a different way of getting me to listen and pay attention."

—Renita J. Weems

Turning to God at crisis points is definitely not unusual. Most patients don't call upon their faith or realize their inner strength until they're really faced with a critical life event, such as a diagnosis of cancer or other terminal illness. Some patients have never thought they had faith. Many have regarded themselves as atheistic. But often the caring that a patient receives when they're facing a serious illness and are surrounded by people who show them true compassion and a Christlike ministry will open their eyes and their hearts, even though they may have turned away from God in the past.

A Beginning Faith

The best part about trust is that we don't have to discover it by ourselves. God is there for the journey, guiding and cheering us along. He found a way to deal with the guilt and shame our first parents felt—a way to welcome Adam and Eve back home again—and He will do the same for each one of us.

The climax of the story of the Garden of Eden is the restoration of intimacy with God. That's what our Creator cares about the most—restored relationship. Spiritual intimacy. God wants to connect each of us to Himself, to the Eternal. That's how we find ultimate peace. It's the only thing that can heal the deepest part of us.

So how do you begin your spiritual journey?

The important thing is to use whatever faith you already have. Get the process started. Jesus' assurance is that even with a mustard seed of faith we can begin a long and wonderful journey.

I have discovered three practical steps that will help you develop an attitude of trust in the Creator.

- ✓ **First, communicate.** Trust grows in an atmosphere of honesty and openness. God has been honest with you. It's time to be honest with Him as well. You can do that in prayer.
- ✓ **Second, listen.** Be open to what God reveals about Himself in His Word, in the Bible.

You've got to get to know someone better in order to trust them, right? So start spending some regular time in study. I suggest you begin with the Gospels (Matthew, Mark, Luke, and John), the accounts of Christ's life on earth. They will provide you a close-up picture of God's character, let you know what He's like. So take time to really drink in each scene, each encounter, each bit of teaching.

✓ **Third, ask.** Start requesting God's help in specific areas of your life. And keep asking. As you continue, you'll begin to learn more and more from the way He answers. His no can be as instructive as His yes. But always ask. That's how you exercise your faith.

LIFESTYLE CHANGES YOU CAN BEGIN TODAY

Always remember that right now you've got faith at least the size of a mustard seed. So use it. Put it to work—and watch your world change.

1. Together time—The key to developing a trust relationship with someone is to spend time together. The same is true with God. Communion between just the two of you is essential to the trust that will lead to health.

2. A quiet place—Do you have a favorite rocking chair, a secluded bench in the park down the street, or a well-worn pew in your church? That may be the perfect meeting place for you and God. Or, for some, it may be in the middle of rush hour with the car windows rolled up and the world on hold. Never miss a

chance to create a "quiet place" for you and God to talk.

3. Scripture—Remember, it's His personal letter to you. And He knows just what you need to hear!

4. Prayer—It can happen anywhere, anytime, and does not depend upon your posture or words. Prayer is talk—honest talk, fearless talk, friend with friend.

5. Books—Take a trip to a Christian bookstore. Wander the aisles and look at everything, especially the books under the "Devotional Reading" sign. Choose three or four of the most interesting and take them to the "reading" chair at the back of the store. Scan a page or two out of each, then select one to buy. We often see God best through the words of His friends.

6. People—Acquainted with someone who seems close to God? Get to know them. Ask questions. Listen. Follow their lead. They just may know the path!

I invite you to start your great adventure with Him—right now in prayer:

"Dear Father, help me to start being honest and straightforward with You. Enable me to begin listening carefully for Your voice. Teach me how I can open up more of my life to You. Build my trust. Nurture my faith. In Your name I pray. Amen."

7

Get Close, Grow Old

The "I" in CREATION Health stands for *Interpersonal Relationships*. Do you value kind words from a close friend? How about a wholehearted hug in hard times? We encounter many of life's greatest joys while sharing hopes and dreams, hurts and hugs with friends. Yet some of these relationships can also be our greatest challenges. People are wonderful—and people are terrible!

That's where the Creator comes in with His basket of "relationship tools." Tools such as grace, love, truth, and time. Tools intended to grow, nurture, and even repair relationships. Tools designed to help us become healthy humans and compassionate friends.

Relationships work best with His tools.

SCIENTIFIC SUPPORT FOR *INTERPERSONAL RELATIONSHIPS*

Did you know that the more friends you have, the less likely you are to catch a cold? That's what Dr. Sheldon Cohen at Carnegie Mellon University has found. Not only that, but if you do come down with a cold, the duration and severity of symptoms will be less if you have lots of social contacts. Conversely, social isolation is devastating to good health. Friends not only increase your capacity for pleasure but will enhance your ability to heal.

In a landmark study reported in the prestigious medical journal, *Lancet,* Dr. David Speigel at Stanford University found that women with breast cancer who participate in psychosocial support groups live significantly longer than breast cancer patients who do not. The finding parallels one reported by investigators at UCLA who discovered that a structured group intervention reduced both mortality and cancer recurrence for the participants.

Sometimes the benefits of a factor are best revealed when examining what happens when it is absent. This is certainly true of social support. Dr. James House reviewed an extensive body of literature in the 1980s that studied a total of 10,000 women. The conclusion was that social isolation will increase your risk of dying from all causes. In the Alameda County study the risk was 2.8 times greater.

GET CLOSE, GROW OLD

What do block parties and low blood pressure have in common? A small town in Rosetta, Pennsylvania, seems to have the answer.

The government discovered that Rosetta, Pennsylvania, was one of the healthiest communities in the country. Wanting to find the reason for its superior health when compared to the rest of the country, they sent a group of investigators there. What they discovered was that its inhabitants were very close-knit. If somebody had a difficulty, the community surrounded them with help. People knew one another, and they would frequently have dinners together. The community's mutual support was way above the norm.

One of the things we're discovering through science is that having a good social support system—deep, personal friendships—can be very beneficial to health.

THE HUMAN HEALING INGREDIENT

In his book *Love and Survival* Dean Ornish, a physician known for his work in reversing heart disease, speaks about the power of love and intimacy. "I am not aware," he writes, "of any other factor in medicine—not diet, not smoking, not exercise, not stress, not genetics, not drugs, not surgery—that has a greater impact on our quality of life, incidence of illness, and the premature death from all causes."

Ornish states that loneliness and isolation increase the likelihood that we may engage in harmful behaviors such as smoking and overeating; that we may get certain diseases or die prematurely; and that we will not fully experience the joy of everyday life. "In short," he observes, "anything that promotes a sense of isolation often leads to illness and suffering. Anything that promotes a sense of love and intimacy, connection and community, is healing." Research from the University of California at Irvine reinforces this point. Its studies indicated that loneliness and lack of emotional support can cause a threefold increase in the odds of being diagnosed with a heart condition. Interestingly, the study also showed that having just one person available for emotional support served to be enough to reduce the risk of heart disease.

ABC News recently carried the story of a small Indian woman on a worldwide hugging tour. Her name is Mata Amritanadamayi, but some have simply dubbed her the "hugging saint." According to best estimates, Mata has hugged more than 20 million people in countries all across the globe. And she shows no signs of slowing down. On her stops in American cities such as New York, Los Angeles, Chicago, Washington, D.C., and Boston, thousands of people line up to be embraced by a complete stranger. When asked where she gets all her energy, she replies simply, "It takes no energy to love. It is easy." Reporter Buck Wolf described his experience with the woman many affectionately call "Amma" or "Mother":

"Here I am, in the deep embrace of a stranger. She folds me into her arms, coos into my ear, and gently kisses my temple . . . 'My son, my son, my son, my son,' she says, rocking me back and forth. 'Love you, love you, love you . . .' I look around me. Here are fellow New Yorkers—rich, educated, and hardened to flimflams. Why do these people wait for hours . . . ?

" 'I'm not religious,' a 28-year-old banker tells me. 'I saw her four years ago in Houston. Now, I just go to her every chance I get. She may be just an old woman who hugs. But there is some beauty in this. Maybe we have to appreciate our need to hug and be hugged—to care for each other.' "

People know when they're cared for—when they're loved. And people who are cared for and loved heal more quickly.

A Heart-to-Heart Companion

God knew the value of relationships from the very beginning. He spent six days filling the earth with plants and creatures of all kinds for Adam to enjoy. But that wasn't enough. Though Adam had a garden paradise abounding with an incredible variety of living things, he needed something more. And God knew just what that was. "The Lord God said, 'It is not good for the man to be alone. I will make a helper suitable for him'" (Genesis 2:18).

Living creatures surrounded Adam, but he was still alone deep inside. His soul held a vacuum. He didn't have the companionship of someone like him—another human being. "So the Lord God caused the man to fall into a deep sleep; and while he was sleeping, he took one of the man's ribs and closed up the place with flesh. Then the Lord God made a woman from the rib he had taken out of the man, and he brought her to the man" (verses 21, 22).

God used Adam's rib to create the first woman. He could have fashioned her from the dust of the ground, as He did Adam. Or He could have made her from nothing. (That's how the Creator usually worked.) But He took something from Adam's chest near his heart to show that this would be a person who would stand by his side. She would be someone who could walk through life with him as a heart-to-heart companion.

Adam recognized his soulmate as soon as he set eyes on her. "And Adam said: 'This is now bone of my bones and flesh of my flesh; she shall be called Woman, because she was taken out of Man'" (verse 23, NKJV).

Bone of my bones, flesh of my flesh. That's what God created in the Garden of Eden. He brought into being human companionship and intimacy. The Creator knew that interpersonal relationships were essential for our health and happiness as human beings.

QUALITY IMPROVEMENT

I've discovered that it's not just the quantity of our relationships, but their *quality* that counts. It's not just how many people we know, how many people we say hi to each day. Rather, it's letting other people really know us. Relationships are most nurturing when we take the time to form that kind of bond.

The quality of our relationships, to a large extent, determines the quality of our lives. The more challenges we face, the more we need other people. One person in a crisis is a tragedy. Two people in a crisis constitute a support group. A sense of belonging makes people feel cared for, loved, and valued. It provides social comfort and a sense of control throughout life's unexpected twists and turns.

> *"One of the finest virtues is generosity—a quality*
> *characteristic of the person who thinks*
> *more highly of others than he does himself."*
> —*Malcolm Maxwell*

Todd Meyer's family became his support group when he underwent a difficult time in his life—cancer. "Before I was diagnosed," he says, "when the doctor told me, 'It looks like lymphoma and we need to do some lab tests to find out for sure,' I was in sort of a state of shock. Because here I'm working at the Walt Disney Memorial Cancer Institute for Florida Hospital doing cancer research, and I'm supposed to be safe from this stuff, you know. But it just doesn't work that way.

"When I told my family that my doctor was talking to me about lymphoma," Todd continues, "it was difficult, although everybody was very supportive. No one took the attitude that this was the end. Instead, people rallied around me and tried to offer support whenever they could. It is very important for family to be involved in healing. We sometimes don't realize it, but we're affected by the people around us."

When family and friends pull together for the ones they love, something remarkable occurs. Grace happens. Healing takes place. It may not always be a physical healing—it may be just emotional or spiritual. But it's healing nevertheless.

I think of an unconscious mother in critical care and not expected to survive. As her children gathered around her, they shared a lot of remorse. "If only I had spent more time with Mom," her youngest son kept saying. "If I just hadn't run away from home . . . I hurt her so badly."

One by one around the group each expressed their regret about things they wished they had said to their mother. As the group prayed together, they asked God to intervene in the situation. Then a miracle occurred. For a short while the mother regained consciousness, and the whole family enjoyed a wonderful time of reconciliation. Everyone said what he or she needed to. The mother brightened up for a considerable period of time, then slipped back into unconsciousness. Shortly thereafter she passed away. Yet she did so with a sense of peace and joy that she hadn't known before. Though the mother did not experience physical healing, her heart and those of her children had emotional healing.

Just as this family found healing in unity, God desires you and me to experience unity with those around us. He wants us not only to be reconciled to Him, but to one another.

INVEST IN OTHERS

The basic picture of a healthy relationship that comes to us out of Eden is that of two people clinging together, two people giving themselves to each other.

In a world full of self-absorbed people, it's easy to develop our own little self-contained universes: *my* personal space, *my* boundaries, *my* needs, *my* limits. We're not nearly as dependent on others as we used to be. And that can sometimes be a good thing. But it has also left us more isolated and self-satisfied. Because we invest less in the relationships that really count, we find ourselves emptier.

> *"We love men not because we like them,*
> *nor because their ways appeal to us, nor even because*
> *they possess some kind of divine spark.*
> *We love every man because God loves him."*
> —*Martin Luther King, Jr.*

The Creator knew that we needed to be understood on the deepest level. That's why He performed the first marriage in the Garden of Eden. He joined Adam and Eve together to become one flesh. God designed them to cleave together, to cling to each other.

Our marriages and friendships need that kind of commitment today. We find healing and nurture only when we invest time and energy—when we invest *ourselves*—in other people. Meaningful relationships can develop only when we open ourselves up to others. Only to the degree that we become honest and transparent before them will we find nurture and healing.

Adam and Eve knew this kind of transparency. The Bible says, "And they were both naked, the man and his wife, and were not ashamed" (Genesis 2:25, NKJV). Such nakedness is much more than two people without clothing. It is two people who are vulnerable before each other, who have nothing to hide.

That's the kind of relationship God established in the garden. In the beginning He made possible a healthy, honest, accepting companionship. And that's still His plan for each one of us today.

"I have loved, and I have been loved.
All the rest is just background music."

—Estelle Ramey

LIFESTYLE CHANGES YOU CAN BEGIN TODAY

Healthy relationships are gifts that keep on giving, producing healing and wholeness for years to come. You can become a giver today.

1. Family—Learn about your family history and prepare a photo storybook of your heritage.

Create a family "coat-of-arms" with symbols that describe you, your parents, and other family members. Best of all, spend personal time with each family member this week.

2. Friends—Nurture quality friendships. But it takes dedicated special time and usually includes food, walks, sports, and conversations about *everything!*

3. Neighbors—Be attentive and friendly to those who live near you. If you have elderly neighbors, offer to chauffer them to the grocery store. Welcome new families with pies, breads, or flowers. Offer to mow and edge their lawns while your neighbors are on vacation.

4. Organizations—Join a local organization in which you can share your skills and develop new friendships. Become a Big Brother or Big Sister. Help build a Habitat for Humanity home. Read to kids at the library. Coach soccer.

5. Church—A church family can easily become the core of your personal support system. Do more than attend—choose to become involved with the service ministries offered at your church. Helping others is one of the best ways to boost your health.

6. Work—Don't neglect the valuable relationships with your coworkers. Learn about them, their families, and their hopes. In the process your work may even become easier!

8

It's All in Your Head

The "O" in CREATION Health stands for *Outlook*. Outlook is a gift you give yourself, the colors with which you paint the world. Some of us leave smudges of gray and dark purple as we frown through the day. That's our choice. Others leave sparkling designs of gold, green, and sky-blue. That's also our decision.

God designed each of us to be different, special, unique, and wonderful. But having a negative outlook is not in His plan. A negative outlook switches off the lights of hope. It changes love to hate and peace to stress.

A positive outlook does just the opposite. It turns on the lights, ignites love, and sets our hearts to dancing. Positive is what He made us to be. Positive like Himself.

SCIENTIFIC SUPPORT FOR OUTLOOK

Attitude is more than simply a state of mind. It can influence how the brain can manage healing. Dr. Richard Davidson at the University of Wisconsin has discovered that people who have a positive attitude have more electrical and metabolic activity on the left side of the brain's prefrontal lobe. This is the side of the brain that, when activated, is associated with greater numbers of natural killer cells—the ones that help us fight viruses and perhaps even cancer. It's not clear which is the chicken and which is the egg, but some studies suggest that simply by thinking positive thoughts you can turn on the side of the brain linked with improved immunity.

Dr. Margaret Kemeny has found that personal expectations are a significant predictor of HIV progression, especially when the person with a pessimistic outlook has experienced loss. The patients in the study had a greater decrease in CD4 T-cells and a greater increase in serum and cell surface activation markers. Exactly how attitude can influence the prognosis of a patient with HIV is not clear. It may somehow trigger changes in the immune system through fear centers in the brain. Or perhaps the negative affect causes the person to give up and ignore options that might improve their health.

IT'S ALL IN YOUR HEAD

We've all heard the phrase "it's all in your head." But new scientific research may be proving it has more truth in it than we ever imagined. The evidence points to a very real correlation between the mind and the body.

> *"The greatest part of our happiness or misery depends on our disposition and not our circumstances."*
> —*George Washington*

"More and more doctors—and patients—recognize that mental states and physical well-being are intimately connected," wrote Michael D. Lemonick in "How Your Mind Can Heal Your Body" (*Time,* Jan. 20, 2003). "An unhealthy body can lead to an unhealthy mind, and an illness of the mind can trigger or worsen diseases in the body. Fixing a problem in one place, moreover, can often help the other."

Depression is proving to be particularly destructive to physical health. "Depression jumps out as an independent risk factor for heart disease," reports Dwight Evans, a professor of psychiatry, medicine, and neuroscience at the University of Pennsylvania. "It may be as bad as cholesterol."

Heart disease isn't the only illness worsened by depression. Those who suffer from cancer, diabetes, epilepsy, and osteoporosis all appear to "run a higher risk of disability or premature death when they are clinically depressed." In fact, 10 percent of diabetic men and 20 percent of diabetic women also have depression—a rate double that of the general population. Depressed diabetic patients were far more likely to have complications, including heart disease, nerve damage, and blindness.

According to studies by Philip Gold and Giovanni Cizza at the National Institute of Mental Health, depressed premenopausal women exhibit a much higher rate of bone loss than those who aren't depressed. An estimated 350,000 women get osteoporosis each year because of depression, says Cizza. Various studies have tied depression to several other diseases, including cancer, Parkinson's disease, epilepsy, stroke, and Alzheimer's.

Just as depression can paralyze our outlook, so can

negative emotions such as anger and fear. A fascinating Duke University study called "Anger Kills" examined the profile of physicians in medical school to determine their anger scale. (In this case, anger wasn't simply being upset at a particular incident—that can happen to anyone. Anger here meant a life orientation, the explosive personality that resents everything. Those physicians high in the anger scale had a greater incidence of heart disease 25 years later.)

Following the September 11, 2001, attacks on the World Trade Center, Jonathan Steinberg, chief of cardiology at New York's St. Luke's-Roosevelt Hospital Center, led a study on New York City's heart patients (see "Our Bodies, Our Fears," *Newsweek,* Feb. 24, 2003). He found that they suffered twice the usual rate of life-threatening heart arrhythmias in the months following the attacks. "Prolonged stress has physiological consequences," Steinberg observes. "These patients experienced potentially fatal events, even though many of them had trouble identifying themselves as unduly fearful."

"The psychological state of fear affects us biologically," said Los Angeles psychiatrist Carole Liberman. "People who are anxious drink and eat more. They have more accidents. They're more likely to get colds or suffer heart attacks."

"Stress," adds Afton Hassett, an expert in psychosomatic illness, "almost always comes out in a bodily symptom."

FROM HELPLESSNESS TO OPTIMISM

Several years ago researcher Martin Sullivan

performed experiments showing that we could teach dogs to become helpless in various situations. Sullivan then applied those same experiments to human beings. He discovered that during the course of our lives we all develop something called learned helplessness.

How do we change this? Sullivan found something called learned optimism—that we could change our outlook so that we could begin to believe that we do have a role in altering our lives. While we can't change other people and some circumstances, we *can* take control of our lives and take small steps toward transforming our outlook, and in turn, our health and wellness.

Earlier in this book I cited Holocaust survivor Viktor Frankl's book *Man's Search for Meaning*. Frankl wrote it after spending two years as a prisoner of war. During that time he concluded: "I have very little liberty from a physical standpoint." But, he said, "I have all the freedom in the world to intellectually frame the experiences that come into my life. . . . We who lived in concentration camps can remember the men who walked through the huts comforting others, giving away their last piece of bread. They may have been few in number, but they offer sufficient proof that everything can be taken from a man but one thing: the last of human freedoms—to choose one's attitude in any given circumstances, to choose one's own way."

We do have a choice—we don't have to become victims. Outlook is not the consequence of what others do to me—*I* am in control of my outlook. Life is the way *I* decide it will be. So I can opt to see the good. I can choose to see the beautiful, to appreciate what surrounds me. My choices alter the way I view life, either improving or distorting my perspective.

> *"We all procrastinate at one time or another.*
> *The most unfortunate procrastination*
> *of all is to put off being happy."*
>
> —*Maureen Mueller*

IN THE JUNGLE, THE QUIET JUNGLE

Believe it or not, these groundbreaking mindbody discoveries have their roots in the Creation story. This part of the story, though, often gets passed over.

Genesis 2:19 describes what happened after God created the animals. "Out of the ground the Lord God formed every beast of the field and every bird of the air, and brought them to Adam" (NKJV).

Try to imagine the scene. Although Adam was a fully developed man, he was also a newborn in a sense. Gazing at all those powerful beasts could have greatly intimidated him. After all, they were some pretty fearsome-looking creatures. But notice what God did. "[He] brought them to Adam to see what he would call them. And whatever Adam called each living creature, that was its name. So Adam gave names to all cattle, to the birds of the air, and to every beast of the field" (verses 19, 20, NKJV).

Isn't this a wonderful touch in the story of Creation? Do you see what God was doing here? He was saying, "Don't be afraid. These are your pets. Give them each a name. They're your playmates."

Adam had an entire zoo to play with, a boundless supply of furry friends.

From the very beginning the Creator sought to instill in Adam a positive outlook on the world around him. He didn't see dangers or enemies—he saw playmates.

A little earlier, the biblical narrative declared that "the Lord God planted a garden eastward in Eden, and there He put the man whom He had formed" (verse 8, NKJV). The Creator placed him in what He called a garden—a beautiful and magnificent one. That really says a lot. God helped Adam view the world as a garden where it was safe to play and safe to grow. He guided him to regard nature as a source of nurture.

In the Garden of Eden the first human being received a wonderful message—play with all your heart, live with all your life, and love with all your being.

It was a positive outlook, a perspective that expects good things. This is another key element in the Genesis story of Creation. And now twenty-first-century research affirms this same principle—that it's our outlook, the way we think about life, that shapes our world. We have to *own* our viewpoint, take responsibility for it. Each of us can change our environment from a jungle into a garden—we can turn beasts into pets.

THINK POSITIVE

Later in the Creation story God gives us a hint as to how to maintain a positive outlook. His instructions come in the form of a warning to Adam and Eve about the tree of knowledge of good and evil. Notice how He presents it: "And the Lord God commanded the man, saying, 'Of every tree of the garden you may freely eat; but of the tree of the knowledge of good and evil you shall not eat' " (verses 16, 17, NKJV).

Fruit trees of every sort filled the Garden of Eden. And God said, "All this is yours to enjoy. There's just one tree—one kind of fruit—that's not good for you."

What's the picture God is reinforcing here? What's the perspective? "Look at all that is good," He is saying. "Keep that in mind. Don't get stuck staring at the bad."

In the New Testament Paul expands on that positive perspective. "And we know that all things work together for good to those who love God," he tells us, "to those who are called according to His purpose" (Romans 8:28, NKJV).

In other words, bad things may happen to us. But God is busy bringing out good in everything. So we shouldn't get stuck in anxiety—we should live in hope.

The opposite of hope is despair or depression. A 15-year study done by Kaiser Permanente, the largest managed health-care organization in the United States, concluded that depressed people utilize health-care services five times more than the normal population. Thus teaching people hopefulness is a way of helping them to overcome depression and, in fact, improve their health.

"People who have hope," says Rebecca Moroose, "people who have a goal, people who have a destiny that they want to see fulfilled will often live longer than those who involute—who curl up and die when they have a serious diagnosis."

In places such as physical therapy clinics up to 80

percent of recovery relates to mental outlook. As one therapist puts it: "Somebody who has suffered an injury and is needing to physically recover—we've got to see the mental part join in. Getting them inspired—it's a lot of work, it's hard, it's difficult. But to see the daily gains that they can make, this is what's going to inspire them mentally to say, 'You know what, I can do this.'"

I've had the benefit of a father who was very optimistic. In fact, he used to say to me that discouragement is the devil's anesthesia when he wants to take your heart out. I believe that hope, on the other hand, is the generic drug of the soul.

FORGIVE YOUR HECKLERS

In many cases choosing hope has a lot to do with letting the past be the past. In the beginning, back in the garden, the Creator modeled an attitude of forgiveness. After all, He'd been wronged. Adam and Eve had eaten the forbidden fruit. They had discounted God's counsel and betrayed His trust in them.

How did the Creator react? Did He turn His back on those who disappointed Him? Did He start plotting against them?

No. He didn't hold a grudge or grow bitter. Instead, He showed Adam and Eve how they could find forgiveness.

That's the second essential component of a positive outlook—forgiveness. You have to be willing to forgive—to let go of the wrongs done to you. Psychologist Loran Toussaint and his colleagues at the Institute for Social Research at the University of

Michigan found that forgiving others had a strong link with better self-reported mental and physical health. Other studies have shown that holding on to hostilities and the resulting stress it produces can weaken the immune system and increase the risk for heart attack. On the other hand, possessing a spirit of forgiveness can actually reduce the same risk.

Herdan Harding tells a story of a baseball player in the Los Angeles Dodgers' minor league system. When something went wrong, the athlete would break or throw bats, seemingly as a way to prevent other people from criticizing him first. Such behavior, though, made him somewhat of a target, particularly to two fans who heckled him on a routine and rigorous basis.

Once, after the batter had struck out, the two young men again began taunting him. The player strode over to the fence where they sat a couple rows back and gestured to them to come down. They weren't so sure they wanted to meet him, but they gathered their courage and went. Instead of being furious, which would have been his typical reaction, he now chose to respond differently. Flipping his bat over, he grabbed it by the barrel, extended the handle to the two men, and said, "Do you guys want a Dodgers' bat?"

After that, they never badgered him again. Attending almost every game, they did nothing but support and encourage him just as loudly as they had previously heckled. It was one of those things that changed the baseball player's life, because he realized that he could choose to do things differently. Not only did it alter his outlook, but it actually had an advantageous transformation on his environment as well.

He may or may not have known it, but this baseball player followed Paul's advice when he forgivingly dealt with the two hecklers. "And be kind to one another, tenderhearted, forgiving one another, even as God in Christ forgave you" (Ephesians 4:32, NKJV). You see, if we hold on to grudges and hurts, then our hearts sicken, our souls shrivel, and eventually our bodies will physically suffer as well.

UNPARALYZE YOUR OUTLOOK

Too often when bad things happen to us and we're in pain we want to blame someone, want to make someone else hurt. What we need to do is to look for a solution. Instead of projecting them onto other people, we need to deal with our own problems. We must stop the blame game and start taking responsibility for our own emotions and behavior.

In His sermon on the mount Jesus commented about people with a compulsion to criticize others: "First remove the plank from your own eye, and then you will see clearly to remove the speck from your brother's eye" (Matthew 7:5, NKJV).

Take the plank out of your own eye. In other words, work on your own issues. Don't blame other people—find a solution. That's the third component in the healthy perspective, even when things get bad.

First, look for the good.

Second, learn to forgive.

And finally, take responsibility.

It's not just what happens to us, it's how we look

at it that counts the most. Our perspective determines our progress—in all kinds of life situations.

"When I'm glad I feel like I'm about to float up in the air, like a butterfly is lifting me from inside."
—Emily Vannoy, age 9

The story of Donna Marini dramatically illustrates this point.

"When I first realized that I was paralyzed and I was going to be in a wheelchair," she remembers, "I was real upset and hurt and felt like somebody owed me—you know, this wasn't fair, why me? Then I realized as time went on that it wasn't going to get much better, so I just needed to accept it. No one was going to beg me to do stuff, so I needed to be the person to continue on with my life and make something, be happy, 'cause you know . . . it's the best that it's going to be."

"Donna had been in a wheelchair for 11 years before she came to see me," Jeannine Chobotar, her physical therapist, remembers. "What really impressed me about her was her outlook on life. Although she was still wheelchair dependent, Donna learned to dress and bathe herself. She made her own food and learned to drive her own car. In fact, she has actually gone back to her profession as a model."

"I didn't think that I'd ever be able to meet a great guy," Donna admits. "But I did and got married. Now I go out and talk to newly injured people and encourage them. Look at me, I tell them. I'm doing fine. Things *will* be OK. You *can* go on."

"After being in a wheelchair for 11 years, it would have been very easy for Donna to have become discouraged, depressed, and maybe even hateful about life," Jeannine observes. "But instead, Donna has taken her situation and become an inspiration to me and to many other people."

"Life is so fragile, as they always say," Donna comments, "and I so appreciate what I have now. And you know, life is not really so bad—it's pretty good. I can still have fun and do things."

A positive outlook can make the difference between recovery and paralysis. And God has given us wonderful promises and assurances that can keep us going, even in the worst of times. Here again are three practical tips on improving your outlook.

First, look for the good in situations and in people.

Second, learn to forgive—don't dwell on the past.

Finally, assume responsibility for your actions, behavior, and emotions.

Do an internal inventory. What kind of attitude have you been carrying with you? Or what attitude do you bring home at night? Take a hard look at your point of view. Does it need some basic adjustments? Could you deal with your problems in a very different way?

I urge you to allow God's positive outlook, created from the very beginning in the garden, to illuminate your mind and heart. Let His perspective sink in today.

LIFESTYLE CHANGES YOU CAN BEGIN TODAY

Healthy relationships are gifts that keep on giving,

producing healing and wholeness for years to come. You can become a giver today.

1. Choose—No one can force you to be bored—or unhappy. You are ultimately in charge of your outlook.

2. Self-talk—How you talk to yourself plays a major part in whether your outlook is positive or negative. If you are telling yourself that you're a valuable person and a success, you will likely become what you hear yourself saying. Compliment yourself on every step of your progress toward CREATION Health.

3. Distraction techniques—Sometimes life seems overwhelming. That's OK. You're in charge! Use a distraction technique to give you some time and distance so you can choose the best response to the situation.

   a. Shift attention: Simply think about something else. Imagine, for example, a piece of warm apple pie with ice cream dripping down the crust. You'll find that while you visualize the pie you have no capacity for whatever negative thoughts were attacking you before. Also you'll be able to plan what to do next.

   b. Make an appointment for later: When negative thoughts chase each other through your mind, make yourself an appointment for later to mull them over. Often things look better away from the spotlight of the moment, and your responses will be wiser.

   c. Write it down: Put it on paper, and the negative thought tends to lose its hold on you.

9

Enrich Your Eating Experience

T he "N" in CREATION Health stands for *Nutrition*. The Creator designed us to get peak performance from the best foods. Then He planted a garden full of them and said, "Enjoy!" We've been reveling in His delights ever since.

The Creator also gave us guidelines for enjoying His goodies. Some foods provide the bursts of energy we need in the morning. Others help us slow down in the evening. Certain ones are great in small quantities and terrible by the plateful. Some bring out flavors while others mask them. The options are many, but the aim is the same. Good nutrition is the process of balancing God's great gifts for full health.

He is the best Chef.

SCIENTIFIC SUPPORT FOR *NUTRITION*

You are what you eat, and that includes your mental well-being. Researchers at Harvard University have discovered that you can adjust serotonin, a brain chemical linked with depression, by varying the amount of carbohydrates in your diet. Not only that, but when you get depressed, the brain triggers a craving for the carbohydrates capable of restoring the serotonin to normal. In other words, food can affect your mood, and your mood can influence which foods you choose.

Of all the nutritional options available, one is guaranteed to improve your health and enable you to live longer—eat less. Dr. Robert Good has conducted research that shows in both animals and humans that if we reduce caloric intake, it will improve just about all aspects of the immune system. Not only that, but illnesses stemming from an unbalanced immune system become easier to manage. No one is certain of why this happens, although the most likely explanations involve a reduction in lifetime exposure to free radicals and an increased desire to exercise. Whenever you reach a point during a meal when you want more but that would call for seconds or thirds, push the plate away. You'll be exactly where you need to be for optimal health.

By eating the right foods, you might be able to lessen your susceptibility to stress. Ultramarathoners are significantly more vulnerable to upper respiratory infection compared with moderate exercisers. Studies have revealed that when marathoners ingest 5-6 percent liquid carbohydrate, it reduces the stress-induced rise in cortisol. The same procedure also blocks some of the immune system changes normally associated with excessive exercise. While more research is needed, it is quite possible that the consumption of carbohydrates may reduce other consequences of stress-induced cortisol production.

ENRICH YOUR EATING EXPERIENCE
Imagine being able to add healthy, quality-filled

years to your life. Consider all the smiles you could share, the new friends you could make, the many lives you could touch. Added years would mean increased opportunities for your own life. Sound too good to be true? It doesn't have to be.

"Lots of times in medicine," says James Rippe, author of the best-selling *Fit Over Forty,* "we forget about the very significant impact of nutrition on good health. The surgeon general's report on nutrition . . . reminds us that eight out of the ten leading causes of death in the United States have a nutritional or alcohol-related component. So nutrition is very, very important in terms of our good health."

And science is constantly confirming this. Research now finds that eating certain foods—fruits and vegetables, whole grains, and plant proteins—can add quality years to your life.

According to a July 15, 2002, article in *Time* magazine, "Should We All Be Vegetarians?" a number of studies have shown that consuming more plant foods reduces the risk for many chronic illnesses, including heart disease, obesity, diabetes, and many cancers, and is likely a factor for a longer, fuller life.

Research presented at the 2002 International Congress on Vegetarian Nutrition indicates that plant-based eating has many healthy benefits. Individuals with diabetes may have fewer complications when consuming more plant foods as well as find it easier to lose weight. Seniors who choose plant-based eating have a lower death rate and use less medication than those who consume more animal foods. And a plant-based diet increases the intake of heart-healthy fats, while lowering saturated fats and cholesterol.

Moderation, balance, and awareness are the key ingredients when choosing plant-based meals. A variety of fruits and vegetables, whole grains, and plant proteins, coupled with the reduction of animal foods, will decrease the risk for most chronic diseases and increase longevity.

> *"It's a giant circle, and food is the key!*
> *Our food choices can affect our emotional health.*
> *Our emotional health definitely affects our*
> *relationships. Our relationships affect our physical*
> *and emotional health. And our*
> *emotional health then affects our food choices!"*
> —Gary Smalley

Rhonda Ringer, a family practice physician, has watched those who incorporate plant-based diets into their lifestyles receive dramatic results. "I have had patients with diabetes, with out-of-control sugars and lipids," she says, "that with healthy nutritional choices and exercise and activity choices have normalized their blood sugars in a very short period of time."

THE CREATOR'S MEAL PLAN

Because the Creator loves us and wants only the best for us, He gave us guidelines for healthy eating. In the Garden of Eden God created an environment in which Adam and Eve could flourish. It was a fascinating, healthy place filled with plants of every description. God blessed the first human couple and established them as stewards of the riches of Creation. To enable them to fulfill their role He provided them with healthy food that would sustain them for their work. "Then God said, 'I give you every seed-bearing plant on the face of the whole earth and every tree that has fruit with seed in it. They will be yours for food" (Genesis 1:29). What did the Creator offer Adam and Eve? A myriad of fruits and vegetables and a wonderful variety of nuts and grains.

But one food God chose not to include in His healthy-eating plan: animal protein. For many years nutritionists believed that meat, poultry, and fish were the essential sources of protein. They assumed that we must have it to have healthy bodies. However, recent studies show that plant protein not only stacks up well against its animal counterpart, but it also provides other healthy benefits. People using plant protein, for example, lose less calcium from the bones. And because plant protein has no cholesterol and little saturated fat, a diet based on plant protein decreases the risk for heart disease.

The United States Healthy People 2010 objectives reflect the growing evidence for the health benefits of eating more plant foods. They define the key to lifelong health as eating more fruits and vegetables, whole grains, and fiber, with moderate amounts of protein and healthy fats.

But the average American consumes a diet high in processed foods and animal products and low in fruits and vegetables, whole grains, and plant proteins. Because the usual American diet typically stresses cholesterol, saturated fats, and calories, it increases our chances of heart disease, diabetes, and cancer. And the latest reports reveal that 64 percent of all American adults are either overweight or obese. But with a few simple changes in what we eat, we can profoundly improve our health and lower our risk for disease.

What are the alternatives to the typical American diet? Include more fruits and vegetables in your meals by having a piece of fruit at breakfast, snacking on raw vegetables instead of crackers or chips, or making salads a part of your dinner. Have whole grains at least three times each day through eating whole-wheat toast at breakfast and brown rice and beans at dinner or adding barley to your favorite vegetable soup. And don't forget nuts, seeds, and soy products. They provide excellent sources of protein without the cholesterol or saturated fats found in animal products. Such foods also have the added benefit of heart-healthy fats and compounds known as phytochemicals. Phytochemicals supply our bodies with the ammunition needed to protect us from most diseases. Try soy milk on your cereal, a small handful of nuts as a snack, or a soy burger the next time you barbecue.

IT'S YOUR CHOICE

God cares about what we put in our bodies. Why? Because it's part of His great plan for us to lead healthy, productive lives. Our Creator seeks to make us whole. And recognizing this makes it just a little easier for us to begin healthy eating habits.

Change is always difficult. Especially when it comes to what we eat. We know that we should consume more fruit, but we'd much rather have a chocolate sundae for dessert. Also we realize that eating less saturated fat and cholesterol is healthier, but we had to work late, so it's much easier to go through the drive-through for supper. Face it, convenience and taste usually win out.

Yes, altering our diet can be tough. But remember, even small adjustments result in big health benefits. Start with something as simple as switching your afternoon snack to one-fourth cup of nuts or seeds. You'll be surprised how easy it will be to then go on to other healthy eating behaviors.

So how can you get motivated to eat healthier foods, and more important, how do you *stay* that way?

Registered dietitians Meredith Luce and Shawn Noseworthy offer these helpful perspectives for choosing healthier foods and maintaining a satisfying, yet balanced, diet.

"Fruits and vegetables have so much color," Luce tells us. "They add so many dimensions to your plate. Color is the key. Not only do we eat with our taste buds, we also eat with our eyes. So think vibrant color whenever you're selecting food. Plant foods—such as fruits and vegetables—naturally have lots of color, which comes from their health-giving phytochemicals. Picking foods with lots of color is one easy step toward healthier eating.

"When you think about it," she points out, "you want taste to be as satisfying as possible, so start with healthy foods you already like. If you don't like bananas, that's OK. Choose a fruit you do enjoy. I encourage eating lots of fruits and vegetables. These are very important not just for nutrition, but also for fiber. In addition, fruits and vegetables have dimension, color, and texture, all of which makes for great mouth appeal.

"Variety is another important aspect of food choice," Luce adds. "It's one of those things you hear a lot from dietitians, and it's very important, because there is no single perfect food. We encourage variety, because each food group and individual food has its own unique combination of nutrients. If we vary what we eat every day, we are guaranteed a variety of nutrients."

What about animal products? Should we avoid using them entirely?

"What we recommend about meat, poultry, and fish," Noseworthy explains, "is to use them less often. Typically we overuse meat, eating more of it than we need. We don't require that much protein, and meat usually contains the cholesterol and saturated fat associated with a higher incidence of heart disease and cancers. Minimize the amount of animal products you consume. When you minimize these foods, you want to maximize your plant foods."

"Plant foods do not have to be boring," Luce stresses. "Great nutrition and enjoyable eating don't have to be bland."

A HEALTHY MOTIVATION

The apostle Paul also had a few things to say about our bodies. He talks about what God made for us as human beings. "Do you not know that your body is the temple of the Holy Spirit who is in you, whom you have from God, and you are not your own? For you were bought at a price; therefore glorify God in your body and in your spirit, which are God's" (1 Corinthians 6:19, 20, NKJV).

This is an extraordinary way of looking at the human body. And yet it's how the Creator views you.

Paul doesn't say that our bodies are the shell that houses the spirit. Instead, he pictures a temple. That's something valuable. Our bodies are temples of the Holy Spirit.

Because of this, we want to take care of them. We desire to honor God by the way we treat our bodies. Why? Because God says that we're that important. And because our health matters to the one who made us and loves us.

As a result, we eat healthfully because we're worth it. Because we're called to something noble and great. It's a motivation that can stick with us in the long run.

A NEW VIEW

Diana Boyce began experiencing this maximum fulfillment after she made changes in her diet. "I knew that as I was getting older," she says, "I was falling into some very unhealthy habits. Having a very large family and a great number of grandchildren, I love to entertain and would cook a lot as well as eat the wrong things. I knew that if I really, really believed in whole-person health, I needed to do something for myself—I had to take action.

"So I began watching the things I ate and had a more balanced diet. I began to pay more attention to what I was eating, when I was eating, and why I was eating. And it began to change me. Soon I felt better. I had energy when I woke up in the morning. When the alarm went off, I didn't just roll over and beg for more sleep. Many times I was awake before the alarm even sounded. I had the energy to do my very active job all day long. My weight even went down until I had lost about 25 pounds. At the same time my cholesterol level dropped dramatically and my skin tone improved. I just felt better about life."

EATING BETTER TO LIVE BETTER

Seventh-day Adventists have been promoting this kind of healthy eating for quite a long time now. Studies clearly demonstrate the difference it makes. Consider, for example, the Adventist Health Study—a major 30-year investigational study on the life spans of Seventh-day Adventists living in southern California. From it we've learned that Adventists, on average, live seven to nine years longer than the general population. Although we do not understand all of the reasons, it *is* clear that nutritional choices play a major role. Plant-based eating or using smaller amounts of animal protein lead to a longer life span and greater health during those additional years.

Looking back to the Garden of Eden, we find the original foods God gave were fruits, vegetables, whole grains, and nuts. Today science has shown us that such foods lower our risk for heart disease, diabetes, high blood pressure, and certain cancers.

Isn't it wonderful that what our Creator originally provided us in the Garden of Eden is just what we need now—in the twenty-first century? Take advantage of His great advice today to live a better, healthier life.

Lifestyle Changes You Can Begin Today

You may be thinking that it's hard to get started, that it's tough making changes in what you eat, that it seems a bit scary. One simple approach to eating healthier uses the model of the three Ms:

1. *Maximize.* Maximize plant foods by choosing whole grains, fruits, vegetables, legumes, and nuts. Don't constantly eat the same things. Maximize variety and color. Experiment. And maximize your taste. Enjoy your food—without this, the changes won't last.

2. *Moderate.* Moderate the amount of food you eat. Eat until you just feel comfortably full and not until you are stuffed. Pay attention to your serving sizes and consider smaller, more frequent meals. Using the food pyramid as a guide (you will find it listed on most food products) is helpful. And moderate any stress when eating—eating should be a blessing and a pleasure.

3. *Minimize.* Minimize saturated fats. Minimize animal protein intake. Minimize refined sugars and even sugar substitutes. And minimize the amount of salt you use. Taste your food before you shake the salt to see if it really needs any.

These guidelines are simple but effective. As you plan your dietary changes you will find plenty of information available on healthy eating. But beware of gimmicks, and remember that there are no quick fixes. The key to a healthy diet, to reduction of disease, and to a longer, fuller life can be found in the garden.

10

Life at Its Best

Improving the quality of our lives—that's what CREATION Health is all about. In the very beginning, in the book of Genesis, God gave us principles that can make all the difference. The CREATION model of health is God's gift to us. He's showing us the way to wholeness—life at its best—and scientific research supports each principle.

So let's buy into that health plan! It's the one with the biggest payback, the best long-term results. But we need to *decide* that we want this kind of life. It won't just drop into our laps or happen by accident. We must deliberately invest our time and energy into adopting such a lifestyle.

Even small decisions in many different areas will make a difference. Choosing to walk outside in the sunshine; choosing to have weekends that truly allow for rest, relaxation, and rejuvenation; choosing to think positively and to drink more water—the list is endless. Your health and well-being are a journey. An old proverb states that the "journey of a thousand miles begins with the first step." Thus the first step on your health journey is **choice.**

Don't forget to **rest.** Take the necessary time to refresh yourself physically. Your body needs an appropriate amount of rest to function optimally, and we all know that the only thing better than a good night's rest is a lot of good nights of rest! Physical refreshing will yield positive results for you mentally and emotionally as well.

Create a healthy **environment** for yourself. Declutter. Take advantage of our world's natural beauty. Get plenty of fresh air. Breathe! Excite your senses with the pleasing look, taste, sound, smell, and feel of nature.

Determine to be physically **active.** You don't need to purchase an expensive gym membership. Just put on your tennis shoes and go for a walk! And as you begin to enjoy that, pick up the pace and challenge your body to do more. You will be pleasantly surprised at how well your body will respond once you let it loose on the open road.

Remember that God should be at the center of everything we do. The pace of our lives—the stresses that we face daily—work against our making healthy choices. To be truly healthy, we need Him. As you make new decisions for your health ask for His help and **trust in His divine power.**

Don't forget that healthy relationships are just as important as a healthy diet. Choose to cultivate satisfying **interpersonal relationships.** Give hugs and smiles. Spend quality time with those you love and who love you.

How's your **outlook?** Are you thinking positive thoughts or is the glass always half empty? Take an inventory of yourself mentally and emotionally. If things aren't so good and you can't seem to find your way through life, seek the aid and advice of those who care and are skilled in helping.

Last but not least, choose to eat healthfully. Drastic changes are not for everyone and are often inappropriate. Anyone, however, can make small, significant changes in their **nutrition.** Go ahead and eat an apple a day. Limit your intake of red meat. "Eat five (servings of fruits and vegetables) to stay alive"!

Let's remember that each positive choice makes the next one easier. As the good results multiply we gain momentum. We start feeling better and looking better. And there will come a time when we wouldn't go back for anything in the world—we wouldn't trade our lifestyle for any amount of money.

God's CREATION Health model is showing us the way. Make that journey, starting right now, with God at your side. Put into practice the principles you've learned. Principles established by God and supported by medical science. You'll be giving a gift to yourself in body, mind, and spirit. And you'll also be offering a gift to your loved ones—those incredibly special people around you.

About Florida Hospital

In 2003, according to the American Hospital Association, Florida Hospital ranked number one in the nation for inpatient admissions—making it the busiest hospital in America. MSNBC calls Florida Hospital "America's Heart Hospital" because it handles more cardiac cases than any other hospital in the United States. Also, it is the largest Medicare provider in the country. *U.S. News and World Report* recognized it as "one of America's best hospitals" in nine clinical specialties.

For nearly 100 years the mission of Florida Hospital has been "to extend the healing ministry of Jesus Christ." Inspired by our strong Adventist heritage of health ministry, we, along with our sister Seventh-day Adventist hospitals, work toward this goal through a commitment to the physical, mental, and spiritual well-being of our patients. This means that we not only treat illness, but also provide the support and education necessary to prevent disease and to help people live life to the fullest as God intended. At Florida Hospital we use Jesus Christ as our ideal model of compassion and care. As a Seventh-day Adventist medical center, we choose to follow His example in treating others "as we would want to be treated."

Lydia Parmele was the first female physician in the state of Florida and the medical founder of Florida Hospital. Her husband, Rufus, provided the management leadership and led the fund-raising efforts that resulted in the opening of the Florida Sanitarium on October 11, 1908. They saw the need for a special health center—a place where people could be sure of the best scientific treatment. But more than that, she envisioned that Florida Hospital would also help patients to learn how to prevent disease through the judicious use of natural remedies.

The Creation-based lifestyle advocated by our founders remains central to all that we do. As we continue to grow and better serve our community, this one goal will remain unchanged: We will serve each patient and friend individually, doing all possible to help each one achieve CREATION Health in body, mind, and spirit.

To learn more about Florida Hospital and to meet Dr. Kellogg and Dr. Parmele, please visit our Web site at www.CREATIONHealth.com. Florida Hospital is a member of the Adventist Health System.

About the Authors

DES CUMMINGS, JR., PH.D.

Des Cummings, Jr., Ph.D., is executive vice president of business development for Florida Hospital and the Florida Division of the Adventist Health System. In this role he gives leadership to the mission, planning, marketing, new business development, and foundations for the 17 Adventist Health System hospitals in central Florida. He earned a Ph.D. degree from Andrews University in leadership and management with emphasis in statistical forecasting. In addition, he holds a Master of Divinity degree and is an ordained minister of the Seventh-day Adventist Church.

Cummings is committed to advancing the healing ministry of Christ in the twenty-first century through strategies that treat the mind, body, and spirit. Motivated by his vision, he helped direct the development of Celebration Health, a showcase hospital in the Disney city of Celebration, Florida. This facility has attracted international attention as a model of health and healing. As a result, Cummings has received invitations to address thousands of health professionals in numerous conferences to present its vision of health.

Not only is he devoted to the concept of empowering patients to take charge of their health, but his wife, Mary Lou, is a health innovator in her own right. She developed Florida Hospital's first breast-care center, the

Women's Center at Celebration Health, and a parish nursing program that currently involves more than 150 churches and 200 nurses in central Florida. Des and Mary Lou have two children, Tracy Beaulieu, an oncology nurse living in Seattle, Washington, and Derek, a senior technology analyst working in Orlando.

MONICA REED, M.D.

Monica P. Reed, Florida Hospital's senior medical officer, oversees the administrative relationship between the hospital and its 2,000 physicians. In her role as an administrative voice for clinical quality and excellence in health care at the institution, she directs clinical performance improvement initiatives, patient safety, and risk management for Florida Hospital's seven campuses.

She received a Bachelor of Science degree from Loma Linda University in 1982, went on to earn her M.D. from Loma Linda's School of Medicine in 1986, and completed postgraduate work in obstetrics and gynecology at White Memorial Medical Center in 1990.

Reed has filled many other roles at Florida Hospital, including medical director for the Celebration Health Center for Women's Medicine, director of the Loch Haven OB/gyn Group, associate director of the Family Practice Residency Program, and medical adviser for the Center for Women's Medicine. In addition, she has served as a medical news reporter.

In 1997 Loma Linda University's Black Alumni Association selected Reed as Alumna of the Year. One year later Loma Linda named her one of its 75 outstanding female alumni. Reed frequently lectures on a variety of women's health issues. In addition, she has edited a pregnancy reference guide, published several magazine and journal articles, and been a columnist for *Women of Spirit*.

Monica is married to Stanton Reed. They have two daughters: Melanie, 10, and Megan, 8.

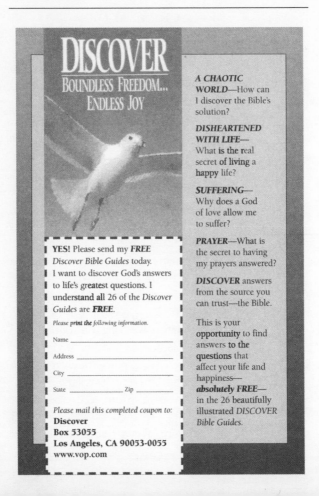